P9-CKH-085

ALL YOU NEED TO KNOW ABOUT

Back Pain

Beat Pain
Increase your Mobility
Know your Options

Compliments of

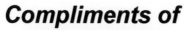
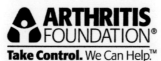

ARTHRITIS FOUNDATION®
Take Control. We Can Help.™

Washington/Alaska Chapter
North Puget Sound Branch

Arthritis Information Line: 1-800-542-0295
www.arthritis.org

ALL YOU NEED TO KNOW ABOUT

Back Pain

Beat Pain

Increase your Mobility

Know your Options

By Mary Anne Dunkin

Chief Medical Editor: John H. Klippel, MD

AN OFFICIAL PUBLICATION
OF THE ARTHRITIS FOUNDATION

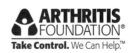
ARTHRITIS FOUNDATION®
Take Control. We Can Help.™

All You Need To Know About Back Pain:
Beat Pain, Increase Your Mobility, Know Your Options

By Mary Anne Dunkin
Chief Medical Editor: John H. Klippel, MD

An Official Publication of the Arthritis Foundation
Copyright 2002
Arthritis Foundation
1330 West Peachtree Street
Atlanta, GA 30309

Library of Congress Card Catalog Number: 2002105663
ISBN: 0-912423-31-5

All rights reserved. No part of this book may be reproduced in any form or by any means without the prior written permission of the publisher, excepting brief quotations used in connection with reviews, written specifically for inclusion in a magazine or newspaper.

Printed in Canada

This book was conceived, designed and produced by the Arthritis Foundation. The mission of the Arthritis Foundation is to improve lives through leadership in the prevention, control and cure of arthritis and related diseases.

Editorial Director: Susan Bernstein
Art Director: Susan Siracusa
Exercise illustrations: Kathryn Born
Medical illustrations: Claudia Grosz

Table of Contents

Chapter 3: Treating Pain With Medications

Chapter 7:
The Importance of a Healthy Lifestyle

Acknowledgements

All You Need To Know About Back Pain is a book written for people who have back pain, as well as for their families and loved ones. While this book should not take the place of the advice and treatment that your physicians and other health-care professionals provide, it may help you better understand your back pain, and may lead you to new solutions for that debilitating pain. Through this deeper knowledge, you can take a more active role in self-managing your condition. This book is published by the Arthritis Foundation, the only national, not-for-profit health agency serving the more than 43 million Americans with arthritis or a related disease.

Special acknowledgements go to the following physicians who reviewed this book for medical accuracy: John H. Klippel, MD, Medical Director of the Arthritis Foundation; David G. Borenstein, MD, Clinical Professor of Medicine, The George Washington University Medical Center, Washington, DC, and author of *Back in Control: A Conventional and Complementary Prescription for Eliminating Back Pain*; Richard A. Deyo, MD, MPH, Professor of Medicine and Health Services, University of Washington; and Randy A. Shelerud, MD, Director of the Spine Center, Mayo Clinic, Rochester, Minn.

This book is written by Mary Anne Dunkin, an experienced health journalist and former Senior Editor of *Arthritis Today* magazine. Ms. Dunkin is also the author of *The Arthritis Foundation's Guide to Managing Your Arthritis*, published by the Arthritis Foundation. The editorial director of the book is Susan Bernstein. The art director and designer of the cover is Susan Siracusa.

The mission of the Arthritis Foundation is to provide leadership in the prevention, control and cure of arthritis and related diseases. This book is inspired by that mission. We hope that its readers will find useful guidance in preventing, controlling and, if possible, curing their back pain.

Foreword

As luck would have it, I am beginning my fourth consecutive week of back pain as I write the foreword to this book – an unbelievable coincidence. I'm not entirely certain what caused the problem in the first place, but I suspect it had something to do with bending over to pull weeds in the garden. My back felt stiff that night, and by the next morning I was having trouble even moving. The pain seemed to be coming from the right side of my lower back, and bending forward or straightening my back produced a sharp pain and caused spasm of the muscles up my spine.

Instead of the symptoms going away after a day or two, as I expected, they have chosen to hang around. I'm now aware of my back constantly, and dread putting on socks, getting my leg in my trousers, rolling over in bed and getting out of a chair. Ignoring the problem doesn't seem to be working, and I'm convinced more than ever of the importance of this book.

Back pain is an enormous problem worldwide affecting millions of people each day, many of whom suffer from chronic back problems leading to disability. The back refers to the lower part of the spinal column, and is made up of bones (called vertebrae), discs that separate the vertebrae, muscles, ligaments, tendons and nerves. Injury to any of these structures as well as a variety of diseases, most commonly arthritis, can lead to acute or chronic back pain. Since the lower back bears the brunt of the weight of the upper body and is needed for bending or twisting movements, back problems can rather quickly take over your life and interfere with almost every activity.

The road to recovery from back pain begins with figuring out what's causing the problem and understanding what you can do about it. Fortunately, most acute back pain is caused by injury with full recovery expected in a matter of days or weeks. There are many things that you can do during this period to relieve the pain. However, it is important that you learn from your episodes of back pain. You can learn to practice preventive measures so that the debilitating back pain doesn't happen again.

Back pain that becomes chronic – long-lasting, whether from injury or disease – is much more of a challenge. Yet there is much that can be done in the way of medications, exercises, preventive behavior and surgery that can be used to treat the signs and symptoms so that you can get on with your life.

This book, *All You Need to Know About Back Pain: Beat Pain, Increase Your Mobility, Know Your Options,* gives you the tools you will need to understand your back pain. In these pages, you will learn about the most common causes of back pain, their many symptoms, how your doctor will make a diagnosis and how you will work with your health-care professional to begin a course of treatment. You will learn about the many drugs, surgical therapies and alternative approaches to treating back pain. Most importantly, you will learn how your actions will impact your health – from exercise to diet to stress and pain management. This book will help you take control of back pain – instead of allowing back pain to take control of your life.

The Arthritis Foundation believes that the actions taken by people with arthritis play a large and important role in determining their outcome. Education, self-management and taking personal responsibility are tools of empowerment and keys to achieving control of back pain. This book, is a practical and clear guide that will hopefully help you achieve a healthier, more fulfilling life.

John H. Klippel, MD
Medical Director
Arthritis Foundation

Introduction

Whatever your walk of life, there is at least one thing you likely share with millions of other Americans – a "bad back."

Back pain is the great equalizer. It affects people of all ages, lifestyles and occupations. Back pain affects an estimated 50 percent to 80 percent of adults at some point in their lives. In any given year, 10 percent of adults (and an increasing number of healthy teenagers) experience back pain or other back symptoms, such as limited mobility or stiffness. Back pain is the most common health complaint, other than the common cold, and surgery to correct or relieve back problems is one of the most common reasons for hospital admissions.

Back pain can range from mildly uncomfortable to excruciating. It can start suddenly, due to an injury or a single action – if, for example, you are injured in a traffic accident or attempt to lift something too heavy. It can come on slowly, sometimes as the result of years of poor posture or age-related changes to the spine. Progressive forms of arthritis, such as ankylosing spondylitis, often start as pain and eventually cause the spine to become rigid.

Back pain and its often lengthy treatments can be costly. Each year, Americans spend an estimated $24 billion on treatments for back pain. That sum doesn't include back pain's other financial costs – such as time missed from work – or, more importantly, the emotional costs of enduring pain and missing out on treasured activities.

Back pain often comes and goes quickly – in many cases, without treatment from a doctor or other health-care professional – but it can linger for weeks, months or even years. Since you are reading this book, your pain most likely falls into the latter category. You'd probably do just about anything to stop the pain. The good news is that there is a lot you can do to stop back pain, or at least to ease it and get on with life despite it.

In this book, we'll look at some of the many causes of back pain as well as the treatments for it, including the ones your doctor can administer or prescribe. You may be surprised to learn that, in many cases, the best weapons aren't surgery or medications. In fact, some of the most effective treatments for your bad back are things you can do yourself – and they don't have to cost a cent.

The key to living comfortably with back pain is you. Yes, there's a lot you can do to ease, stop and even prevent back pain. This book can help you by showing you what to do and how to do it.

chapter 1:

Why Backs Go Bad

Although millions of people experience back pain, most never know precisely what causes it. The good news is that, in most cases, knowing the exact cause of pain isn't necessary to get good treatment results.

Still, to understand why the back is so vulnerable and the kinds of things that can go wrong, it first helps to understand what the back is.

Let's Talk Back

When most people mention their back, what they actually are referring to is their spine. The spine runs from the base of your skull down the length of your back, going all the way down to your pelvis. It is composed of 33 spool-shaped bones called *vertebrae*, each about an inch thick and stacked one upon another.

Each of the vertebrae consists of several parts:

The **body** – the main area of weight bearing.

The **lamina** – the lining of the hole (spinal canal) through which the spinal cord runs.

The **spinous process** – the bony protrusions ("bumps") you feel when you run your hand down your back.

The **transverse processes** – a pair of protrusions on either side of the vertebrae to which the back muscles attach.

The **facets**, two pairs of protrusions where the vertebrae connect to one another, including:

The **superior articulate facets**, which face upward.

The **inferior articular facets**, which face downward.

[See figure page 15.]

The connection points between the vertebrae are referred to as **facet joints**. The facet joints keep the spine aligned as it moves. Similar to other joints in the body, such as the hips or knees, the facet joints are lined with a smooth membrane called the **synovium**. This membrane produces a viscous or thick, slippery fluid called synovial fluid, which lubricates the joints. In some cases, the synovium can become inflamed, causing pain. In other cases, the synovial fluid may lose its thick, slippery quality, causing stiffness.

Located between the individual vertebrae are **discs**, which serve as cushions or shock absorbers between the bones. Each disc is about the size and shape of a flattened doughnut hole and consists of two parts: a strong outer cover called the **annulus fibrosis** and a "jelly filling" called the **nucleus pulposis**.

Because discs don't have a blood supply, they depend on the muscles and other nearby tissues for nourishment. When you lie down and sleep, discs absorb fluid from surrounding tissues and expand. Once you stand up and get moving, the discs squeeze out fluid, causing them to compress. In fact, after a day's activities, compression of the discs can cause you to be an inch shorter than when you woke up that morning.

Although the spine is a continuous structure, it is often described as if it were five separate units. These units are the five different sections of the spine:

1. The **cervical spine** – the neck and upper back, composed of the seven vertebrae closest to the skull. The cervical spine supports the weight and movement of your head and protects the nerves exiting your brain.

2. The **lumbar spine** – the lower back, composed of five vertebrae. The lumbar spine supports the majority of your body's weight.

3. The **thoracic spine** – the middle back, made up of the 12 vertebrae in between the cervical and lumbar spine.

4. The **sacrum** – the base of the spine that attaches to the pelvis, composed of five vertebrae fused (joined together) as one solid unit.

5. The **coccyx** – the "tailbone" located below the sacrum, composed of four fused vertebrae.

Running through the center of the spinal column – from just above the sacrum to the brain – and protected by it is the **spinal cord**, a bundle of nerve cells and fibers about as big around as a personal computer cable or first-grade pencil. The spinal cord transmits electrical signals back and forth between the brain and the rest of the body. It conducts this transmission via 31 pairs of smaller nerve bundles that branch off the spinal cord and exit the column between the vertebrae. Through this transmission, signals from the brain tell the arms, legs and other body parts to move; the brain also translates signals transmitted from other parts of the body as sensations, including pain.

The opening through which the spinal cord passes through the spinal column is the **spinal canal**. Surrounding the cord within the canal is a liquid called cerebrospinal (meaning a combination of brain and spine) fluid, which helps cushion and protect the spinal cord.

Supporting the spine while providing it flexibility are **ligaments** (tough bands of connective tissue that attach bone to bone) and muscles. Two main ligaments that can play a role in back pain are the anterior longitudinal and posterior longitudinal ligaments, which run the full length of the back and hold together all of the spine's components. These two ligaments are key in controlling the motion of the spine, while allowing flexibility.

The two main muscle groups involved in back function are the **extensors** and the **flexors**. Extensors include many muscles that attach to the spine and work together to hold your back straight while enabling you to extend or arch it. The flexors, located at the front of your body, include your abdominal and hip muscles. The flexors attach at your lumbar spine and enable you to bend forward. Other muscles allow you to twist or rotate your spine. [See figure page 15.]

What's Behind Your Pain

Back problems can have many origins – some having to do with the spine itself, others seemingly unrelated. Furthermore, problems in the back can show up elsewhere in the body – as a headache, shoulder pain, numb or tingling leg, or even constipation.

The most common causes of low back pain are mechanical disorders of the lower spine. Any back pain can be classified as mechanical if physical activity makes it worse and rest makes it better. The most common mechanical cause of back pain is probably degenerative disc disease (the breakdown of the cushions between the vertebrae), but a variety of problems – arthritis, sprains, strains or even tumors – can cause mechanical symptoms.

For the purposes of this book, we have divided the causes of arthritis into three categories: mechanical causes, disease-related causes and other causes. Keep in mind, however, that the categories can overlap. Few fit neatly into one category.

MECHANICAL CAUSES

As you age, the discs that cushion the moving vertebrae weaken and become smaller, losing much of their ability to cushion. This condition is called degenerative disc disease. Degenerative disc disease typically doesn't cause pain until you perform a strenuous activity that you're not in shape to do.

Degenerative disc disease is probably the most common mechanical cause of back pain, but there are many are others. Here are some of the most common.

Sprains. When ligaments in the back are torn – usually from a sudden injury – the result can be pain. The pain of a sprain can be mild or severe, localized to one spot in the back or more generalized all over your back and in nearby areas of the body.

Spasms. Sometimes overworked muscles of the back (and elsewhere) go into spasm – painful, involuntary contraction, similar to a charley horse (a cramp, usually occurring in the calf muscle). While spasms are painful, they are the body's way of protecting itself from the underlying problem. When muscles are in spasm, they become painful and rigid, so that you temporarily are unable to use or damage them further.

Ruptured or herniated discs. When discs are weakened, the hard outer covering can rupture, allowing the squishy center to bulge out and put pressure on nearby nerves.

Poor posture. Slumping the shoulders or hunching over your desk can place abnormal pressures on the spine and lead to back pain. On the other end of the spectrum, the military stance – shoulders back, chest out – can aggravate back pain in people with such problems as herniated or degenerative discs, or arthritis of the spine.

Coccydynia. Literally translated as pain in the coccyx, or tailbone, coccydynia is usually the result of trauma, typically caused by falling directly onto your buttocks. Such trauma can occur if you slip on a slick surface, such as an icy sidewalk or a waxed supermarket floor.

Facet syndrome. Facet syndrome is inflammation of one or more of the facet joints where the vertebrae connect to one another. The condition can be painful, and many patients describe the pain as a deep, persistent ache.

Muscle tension. When some people are stressed out or tense, they feel pain in the muscles of the neck, shoulders and upper back. This pain can be very intense and can worsen if not addressed.

DISEASE-RELATED CAUSES

Though back pain is more likely to be the result of purely mechanical causes than underlying disease, certain diseases can play a role in back pain for a significant number of people. It's important to note that virtually any disease can cause mechanical symptoms – that is, symptoms that worsen with use and improve with rest. Many different diseases can affect the back. Among the most common are the collection of diseases referred to as **arthritis**.

Arthritis

Literally meaning joint inflammation, arthritis is actually a group of more than 100 diseases that affect the joints. Because the spine is made up of 48 joints, it is commonly affected by arthritis. Although almost any form of arthritis can affect the spine, the following types are most commonly involved:

Osteoarthritis. The most common form of arthritis, osteoarthritis (often abbreviated as OA) grows increasingly common as we age. Sometimes referred to as degenerative arthritis, OA occurs when joint cartilage (the tough, smooth connective tissue that covers the ends of the bones where they meet) breaks down. As the cartilage breaks down, the bone at the end of the joint can thicken and develop bony growths called **spurs**. This process can affect virtually any joint, but the facet joints (those joints where the vertebrae connect to one another) at the lumbar spine are among those commonly affected.

Osteoarthritis of the spine may or may not be painful. In some people, it causes limited motion and a stiff back that is worst after awakening in the morning and gradually improves through the day. In others, the pain and stiffness may be worse at the end of the day.

Ankylosing spondylitis. Ankylosing spondylitis is a rare form of arthritis that primarily affects the spine, causing inflammation and stiffening of the joints or ligaments of the spine. It typically begins in the sacroiliac joints and lower spine and may progress upward to the neck. In severe cases of ankylosing spondylitis, the spine can become fused in a rigid stooped or upright position. Ankylosing spondylitis is one of a group of conditions referred to as spondyloarthropathies (that is, arthritis that affects the spine.)

Other spondyloarthropathies. At least three other diseases fall into the category of spondyloarthropathies. They are:

1. **Reactive arthritis** – a form of arthritis that often follows an infection of the bowel or genital/urinary tract.
2. **Psoriatic arthritis** – a form of arthritis that occurs along with psoriasis (skin disease characterized by scaly, flaky patches).
3. **Arthritis with inflammatory bowel disease** – a form of arthritis that is accompanied by chronic inflammation of the intestine.

In addition to their effects on the joints of the spine, all spondyloarthropathies can affect the joints of the arms, legs, feet and hands.

Rheumatoid arthritis. Joints of the spine – particularly those of the cervical spine – are among many that can be affected by rheumatoid arthritis (abbreviated as RA), a form of the disease that causes pain, inflammation, joint damage and deformity. RA is believed to be an autoimmune disease, one that occurs when the body's immune system attacks and damages healthy tissue. In RA, the primary target of that attack is the synovium, the smooth membrane that lines the joints. It is one of the more rare causes of back pain.

Other diseases and conditions

Other diseases and medical conditions – some related to arthritis and some not – that can cause pain and other problems in the back include the following:

Osteoporosis – The spine is one of the most common sites of osteoporosis, or thinning bones, which can occur with aging, inactivity, a low-calcium diet or long-term use of glucocorticoid medications. The inner spongy bone and more solid outer portion of the vertebrae are both affected, becoming porous. The weakened vertebrae can break – an injury called a compression fracture – and lose about one-half of their height. In most cases, compression fractures are painful; in some cases, the pain is severe. Usually, the pain resolves within a few weeks, but for some people, it is long-lasting.

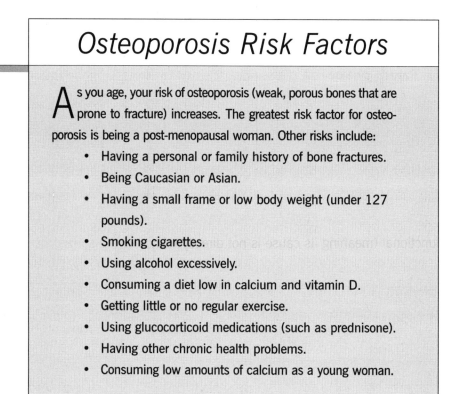

Osteoporosis Risk Factors

As you age, your risk of osteoporosis (weak, porous bones that are prone to fracture) increases. The greatest risk factor for osteoporosis is being a post-menopausal woman. Other risks include:

- Having a personal or family history of bone fractures.
- Being Caucasian or Asian.
- Having a small frame or low body weight (under 127 pounds).
- Smoking cigarettes.
- Using alcohol excessively.
- Consuming a diet low in calcium and vitamin D.
- Getting little or no regular exercise.
- Using glucocorticoid medications (such as prednisone).
- Having other chronic health problems.
- Consuming low amounts of calcium as a young woman.

Spinal stenosis – Literally meaning "spinal narrowing," spinal stenosis can occur when osteoarthritic changes lead to bony overgrowth of the vertebrae and thickening of the ligaments. If significant overgrowth occurs, it can cause the spinal column to narrow and press on the nerves housed within. Because the affected nerves have many functions, the condition may cause diverse problems in the lower body, including back pain, pain or numbness in the legs, constipation or urinary incontinence.

Diffuse Idiopathic Skeletal Hypertosis (DISH) — A disorder that causes excess bone to grow between the vertebrae, DISH is most common in older men. In DISH, the vertebrae from the neck to the lower back usually are affected, causing spinal stiffness. DISH usually does not cause much pain.

Paget's disease — A disease characterized by excessive bone breakdown followed by abnormal formation. The abnormally formed bone is not as strong as healthy bone and, as a result, can break easily. Paget's disease can affect the vertebrae, causing them to become enlarged, but weakened.

Scoliosis — Instead of running straight up the center of the back, a spine with scoliosis twists to one side. Scoliosis can be classified as true (meaning it has to do with abnormal development of the spine) or functional (meaning its cause is not directly related to the spine).

Functional scoliosis may occur when a discrepancy in leg length causes the pelvis to tilt to one side to compensate. The tilting pelvis, in turn, causes the spine to curve. The cause of true scoliosis is largely unknown, although doctors suspect that it may be the result of imbalanced growth in childhood. If one side of a child's body grows faster than the other, it can cause the two sides of the spine to be unbalanced and the soft tissues on the affected side to shorten. Scoliosis generally does not cause back pain, but it can present a problem with movement and normal back function.

Kyphosis — An abnormal forward curvature of the upper spine, kyphosis is sometimes referred to as **hunchback** or a dowager's hump. In children and adolescents, the condition is uncommon, but it can be inherited or caused by infection or injury. In adults, the most common cause is osteoporosis.

Spondylolysis – If the facet joints that connect the vertebrae are weak or damaged due to trauma or an inborn defect, the vertebrae may detach from one another – a condition called **spondylolysis**, which may or may not be painful. If the affected vertebrae move out of alignment, the result is a condition of a similar name – **spondylolisthesis**. Spondylolisthesis can cause back pain or pressure on the nerves as they exit the spine.

Tumors – In rare cases, tumors – either malignant (cancerous) or benign (not cancerous) – affect the vertebrae or other tissues near the spine, causing back pain.

Infections – Infrequently, back pain can be caused by infection that travels through the bloodstream to the spine. The original site of infection can be virtually anywhere in or on the body. One infection-related cause of back pain is **discitis**, or inflammation of the discs.

Fibromyalgia – An arthritis-related condition, fibromyalgia is a syndrome of fatigue, which can be debilitating, and chronic muscle pain over a large part of the body. The lower back is a common site of fibromyalgia pain.

Other causes

Other causes of back pain are numerous. Some common causes of back pain that aren't directly related to the spine include the following:

Arachnoiditis – The scarring of tissue surrounding the spinal nerve roots (where the nerves exit the spine between the vertebrae), arachnoiditis can cause pain, numbness and tingling in the legs. The most common cause of the scarring is prior back surgery.

Obesity – Excess body weight, particularly in the abdomen, causes strain on back muscles, which must work harder to counteract the downward pull of that weight to keep the spine upright.

Pregnancy – Pregnancy, obviously, can cause a quick increase in weight in the abdomen – probably the worst place to carry excess weight, as far as the lower back is concerned. Pregnancy also stretches and weakens the muscles of the abdomen that help support the spine, taking a further toll on your aching back.

Kidney stones or kidney infections – The kidneys' location in the lower back makes them a possible source of back pain. Both kidney infection and kidney stones can cause pain – sometimes intense and severe – that may be felt in the back.

Endometriosis – When endometrial tissue (the tissue that lines the uterus) leaves the uterus and deposits on other organs and structures, it can swell and cause pain, a condition called endometriosis. This condition occurs or worsens around menstruation. The pain of endometriosis usually is felt in the abdomen and lower back.

Aortic aneurysms – In rare cases, the aorta (the body's main artery that originates at the heart and runs down the body just in front of the spine) develops an aneurysm, a balloon-like swelling in the artery's muscular wall. If the wall ruptures or causes compression of the blood vessels that run off it, the result can be pain that is felt in the chest, abdomen and/or lower back. This is a serious situation that requires immediate medical attention and, usually, surgery.

Stress – Many cases of back pain are believed to be related to psychological causes. Even if emotions aren't directly involved in back pain, they certainly play a role in its severity and your response to it. Stress and tension can cause muscle contractions that can lead to or worsen pain. Depression can make pain more bothersome and more persistent. It's important that people seek help for depression and find ways to control their stress. We'll talk more about controlling stress in Chapter 9.

Back Pain: The Long and Short of It

(Acute vs. chronic pain)

While the pain you experience from a day of unaccustomed activity may resolve, never to return, other pain may come and go or, even worse, come and stay – unless you take action to change what's causing or perpetuating your pain.

Just as back pain can be divided into general categories based on cause, it can be divided into three categories based on how long it lasts. Treatment for severe, short-term pain may differ significantly from treatment for pain that goes on and on.

Here are the three categories based on duration of pain:

1. **Acute** – Pain that comes on rapidly and lasts about one to seven days. Acute pain can be mild to severe. It is the most common type of back pain.

2. **Subacute** – Pain that lasts more than a week and possibly as long as a few months. Approximately 10 percent to 20 percent of cases can be classified as subacute.

3. **Chronic** – Long-term pain lasting more than three months. Chronic pain can range from mild to severe. Fortunately, it is the least common type of back pain, representing about 5 percent to 10 percent of cases.

In Chapter 2, we'll take a look at some of the symptoms of the main causes of back pain and discuss how you and your doctor can identify the problem that underlies your pain. Then, we'll explore some of the many ways you can help relieve your pain and permanently prevent its return.

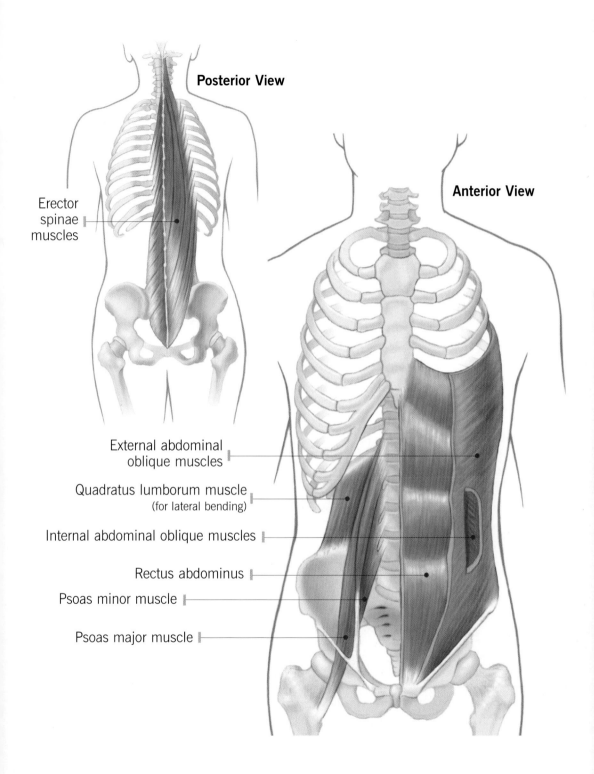

Posterior View

Anterior View

Erector
spine
muscles

External abdominal
oblique muscles

Quadratus lumborum muscle
(for lateral bending)

Internal abdominal oblique muscles

Rectus abdominus

Psoas minor muscle

Psoas major muscle

What Is Your Back?

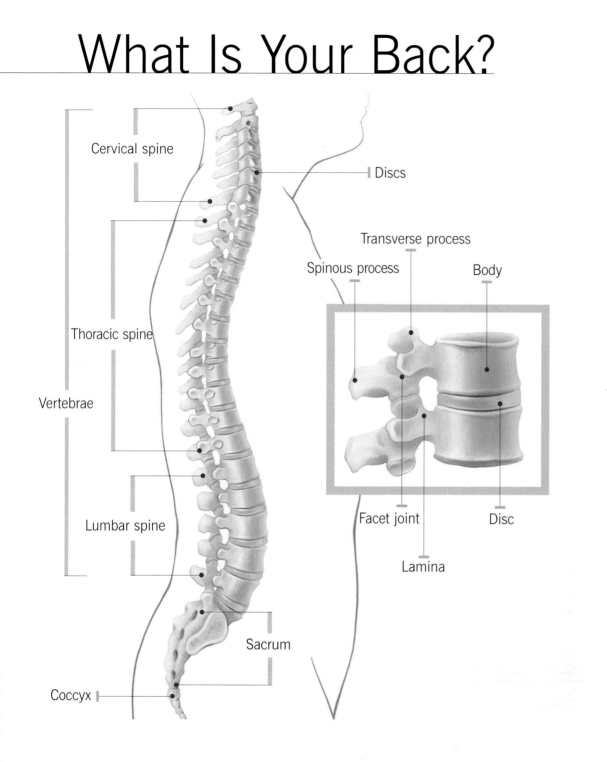

Cervical spine

Thoracic spine

Vertebrae

Lumbar spine

Sacrum

Coccyx

Discs

Transverse process

Spinous process

Body

Facet joint

Disc

Lamina

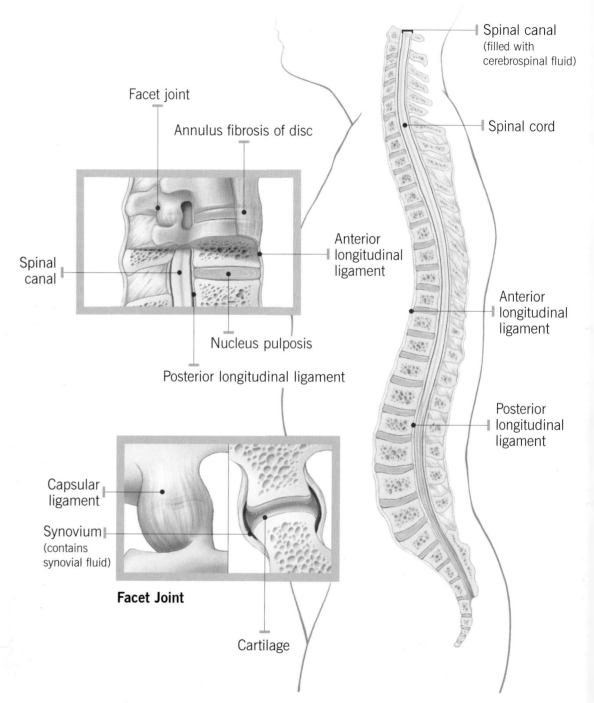

Facet joint

Annulus fibrosis of disc

Spinal canal

Anterior longitudinal ligament

Nucleus pulposis

Posterior longitudinal ligament

Capsular ligament

Synovium (contains synovial fluid)

Facet Joint

Cartilage

Spinal canal (filled with cerebrospinal fluid)

Spinal cord

Anterior longitudinal ligament

Posterior longitudinal ligament

Types of Back Pain

Type	Pain	Duration	% of Cases
Acute	mild to severe	1-7 days	About 80
Subacute	usually mild	7 days to 7 weeks	10 to 20
Chronic	mild to severe and long-term	more than 3 months	5 to 10

A note about the illustration

The preceding foldout illustration shows the many components of the back itself, components you learned about in Chapter 1. As you can see by looking at the illustration, the back consists of many moving parts and soft tissues that can become injured or inflamed, causing anything from acute to chronic pain (see the chart above). This illustration is meant to help you locate some of the areas of the back where your pain is located, and to better understand the diagnosis your doctor will provide. We have included close-up illustrations of the facet joints and the vertebrae to further explain how these amazing constructions work to help your back move in many different directions.

In Chapter 2, you will learn about the many methods your doctor can use to diagnose the probable cause of your back pain, and what symptoms are clues to what causes. Please refer back to this full-color foldout illustration as you read through the book and notice references to parts of the spine and back.

Back Pain: An Equal-Opportunity (and Costly) Offender

Back pain affects people of all ages, lifestyles and occupations. Back pain affects an estimated 50 percent to 80 percent of adults at some point in their lives.

- In any given year, 10 percent of adults (and an increasing number of healthy teenagers) experience back pain or other back symptoms, such as limited mobility or stiffness.

- Back pain is the second most common reason for a visit to a primary-care doctor.

- While back pain is widespread, it is highly treatable. Approximately half of the people who experience back pain will find relief within two weeks. About 90 percent of people with back pain find relief within three months of treatment.

- About five to 10 percent of back pain cases become chronic, or long-lasting, requiring long-term treatment and self-management strategies to control pain.

- Each year, Americans spend an estimated $24 billion on various treatments for back pain.

- According to the Centers for Disease Control, back injuries account for nearly 20% of all injuries and illnesses in the workplace. Back injuries cost an estimated $20 to $50 billion per year in health-care costs and other expenditures and cost American industry $10 to $14 billion in workers' compensation costs and about 100-million lost workdays annually.

- Only a small percentage of all serious back injuries are true sprains, strains or fractures. Most are the result of degeneration of the spine caused by aging and overuse.

- Back pain often affects young, active people. Most back injuries occur among people between the ages of 24 and 40. Younger adults with back pain are more likely to be experiencing a disc-related problem; older adults with back pain are more likely to be experiencing osteoarthritis or similar degenerative joint diseases.

- In the United States, there are nearly 200,000 people living with a spinal-cord injury-related disability. However, most back pain or back injuries do not result in permanent damage or paralysis.

chapter 2:

Oh, My Aching: Diagnosing Back Pain

In the majority of cases, back pain resolves with time – with or without treatment. In most cases, simple do-it-yourself treatments may be all that's needed to help the healing process along. However, because back pain can be a symptom of a serious problem that requires medical attention, it's best to see a physician immediately about pain that occurs after a severe fall or injury, doesn't improve when you lie on your back or is accompanied by one of the following:

- Weakness, pain or numbness in one or both of your legs;
- Fever or unintentional weight loss; or
- Pain or difficulty when urinating.

In those cases, a specific diagnosis and prompt, appropriate treatment may be necessary.

Which Doctor Should You See?

Aside from back injuries that require a trip to the emergency room, most back problems can be evaluated by your primary-care physician.

Depending on the specific symptoms and their severity, however, you may need to see or have your primary-care physician refer you to one of the following specialists. (Note: If you don't have a primary-care physician or a "general-practice doctor," you may wish to consult your health plan or the Web site of the American Academy of Family Physicians, www.familydoctor.org.)

Rheumatologist – a medical doctor (MD) or osteopathic physician (DO) who is specially trained to diagnose and treat the many forms of arthritis and related conditions, including osteoarthritis, ankylosing spondylitis, fibromyalgia, rheumatoid arthritis and osteoporosis – all of which can have back pain as a possible symptom.

If necessary, your doctor can refer you to a rheumatologist. In some cases, your health insurance may dictate the rheumatologist you will see. Another way to find a reputable rheumatologist is by contacting your local Arthritis Foundation chapter for a list of doctors in your area. You can locate your chapter by calling 800/283-7800 or by logging on to www.arthritis.org. You can also ask family, friends or coworkers for recommendations, or check the Web site of the American College of Rheumatology, www.rheumatology.org, which maintains a listing of rheumatologists by state.

Physiatrist (rehabilitation doctor) – a medical doctor who specializes in problems of the muscles and bones. Physiatrists do not perform surgery and although they are licensed to prescribe medication, they focus more on a non-medication rehabilitation approach to back pain and other musculoskeletal problems. Physiatrists are among the most commonly seen and recommended specialists for treating back pain. To learn more about physiatry or to locate a physiatrist in your area, visit the Web site of the American Academy of Physical Medicine and Rehabilitation at www.aapmr.org.

Osteopathic physician – a doctor who has been trained to perform hands-on manipulative treatments, with an emphasis on the musculoskeletal system. The training for an osteopathic physician (DO) otherwise is almost identical to that of an MD. More than one-half of DOs practice in primary-care fields such as family medicine, pediatrics or internal medicine; however, DOs may specialize in different fields, just as MDs do. Many osteopathic physicians specialize in rheumatology, and because of their emphasis on the musculoskeletal system, they may be especially qualified to treat problems of the spine and supporting structures.

To find an osteopathic physician in your area, contact your state osteopathic medical association. Contact information for state associations, along with physician listings for some states, is available on the American Osteopathic Association's Web site, www.aoa.net.org.

Neurologist – a doctor who has advanced training in diagnosing and treating problems related to the nervous system. In cases where the suspected cause of back pain is nerve damage or compression of the nerve roots (through spinal stenosis, for example, or a herniated disc), you may wish to have your primary-care doctor refer you to a neurologist. A neurologist can perform diagnostic tests (see "Nerve Tests" on page 31) to determine the cause of back pain and may treat problems in which structures in the spine impinge on nerves. To learn more about neurology or to find the name of a neurologist in your area, visit the American Academy of Neurology Web site at www.aan.com.

Orthopaedic surgeon – a surgeon who is trained to treat diseases of and injuries to the musculoskeletal system. An orthopaedic surgeon may treat back-related problems, including, but not limited to, spinal stenosis, osteoporotic fractures, scoliosis or herniated discs.

Orthopaedic surgery, as the name suggests, focuses on using surgery to treat medical problems, but it also incorporates the use of medications. To locate an orthopaedic surgeon in your area, speak with your doctor or check out the American Academy of Orthopaedic Surgeons' Web site, www.aaos.org, which allows you to search for a doctor by name or location.

Neurosurgeon – a doctor who has specialty training in the surgical treatment of problems related to the nervous system, including lumbar spinal stenosis and other conditions involving the spine. If your condition warrants treatment by a neurosurgeon, your primary-care physician or neurologist (if you have seen one) can refer you to one. For more information about neurosurgery, check out the Web site of the American Association of Neurological Surgeons/Congress of Neurological Surgeons at www.neurosurgery.org.

Making a Diagnosis

Regardless of the type of physician you see initially, the process of making a diagnosis probably will be similar, involving the following three components.

MEDICAL HISTORY

Back problems present differently – some come on slowly and progress gradually, while others hit you suddenly, making it difficult to stand, sit or do anything without pain. Some are confined to the back, while others are accompanied by other symptoms, such as tingling in or numbness of a leg. (For a sample list of back problems and some of their characteristic symptoms, see page 32.) Your doctor can determine a lot by your description of the problem along with when and how it started, what makes it better and what makes it worse. For example, is it painful when you are resting and at night when you are sleeping, or is it only painful when you are up and active?

Other clues to what's wrong may be found in your medical history. For example, your doctor may ask you questions about your past medical problems, such as, "Have you ever suffered a back injury? Have you had pain or swelling in other joints? Have you ever had cancer? Have you had unexplained weight loss?" Or your doctor might ask you questions about the medical condition of members of your family, such as, "Do you have a close family member with back problems or arthritis?"

Your doctor may also ask questions about your work and lifestyle habits. For example, do you spend a lot of your time sitting at a desk – or on the sofa? Do you exercise regularly, and if so, what type of exercise do you do? Do you smoke, and if so, how much?

Making a note of symptoms and other information you would like to share with your doctor can help you make the most of your time with him or her. For some important points to consider when it comes time for your medical evaluation, see "What To Tell Your Doctor" on page 25.

For your convenience, consider using a journal to keep track of your medical visits, symptoms, experiences, drugs, treatments and other important information. Information about where to procure ready-made health journals is included in the "Resources" section at the end of this book.

PHYSICAL EXAM

Aside from the medical history, the physical exam may provide your doctor the most important clues about the cause of your pain. During

What To Tell Your Doctor

Among the most important clues to a correct diagnosis are the ones you give your doctor. Think about these points before your appointment. Make notes, if it helps you remember, so you'll be prepared to answer your doctor's questions. Note before your appointment:

- When the pain started.
- What the pain feels like.
- How long the pain lasts.
- The time of day the pain is worst.
- Other symptoms you've noticed.
- Other medical conditions you have.
- Childhood illnesses you've had.
- Adult illnesses you've had.
- Surgeries you've had.
- Injuries you've had.
- Lifestyle habits (bad and good).
- Medical conditions your family members have had.

the exam, your doctor will check your posture and look for such problems as curvature of the spine.

Your doctor may ask you to stand and walk to determine if back pain is affecting your gait (the manner in which you walk) or if an awkward gait (perhaps due to leg-length discrepancy or arthritis in the knee or hip) may be contributing to your back pain.

He or she may ask you to move, bend and change positions to see if a particular activity or position makes your pain worse. Some causes of pain may be associated with sitting or standing or other positions or activities. Some are unaffected by position or activity. (For some examples, see "Symptoms of Back Problems" on page 32.)

The doctor may press on different parts of your body – even parts where you may not be aware of pain – to check for **tender points** (tender, painful areas that are characteristic of fibromyalgia – see page 36) and **trigger points** (areas of the body that, when pressed, cause pain elsewhere) and to locate the source of your pain.

Your doctor may test your reflexes by tapping your knee or ankle with a rubber hammer, because slowed or heightened reflexes might suggest nerve problems.

The doctor may also assess your problem through one or more of these noninvasive tests, as part of the physical exam:

Lower body nerve evaluation. By running a device called a pinwheel along your skin, from your hips to your feet, your doctor can check for any areas that are either abnormally sensitive – or insensitive – to stimulus, which would suggest possible nerve involvement in the lower spine.

Muscle-strength evaluation. By checking the strength of the different muscle groups in your lower body, your doctor can detect possible nerve problems. Because different nerves supply different muscle groups, a weakened muscle group may suggest damage to the nerve that supplies that group of muscles.

Sciatic nerve stretch test. By raising your legs one at a time (while you extend and relax them) as you lie flat on a table, your doctor can determine whether stretching the sciatic nerve (the nerve that goes from your back into your legs) causes pain, suggesting possible nerve-root involvement.

MEDICAL TESTS

Depending on the findings of the medical history and physical exam, your doctor may conduct medical tests to help make or confirm a diagnosis. Following are some of the tests most commonly used in diagnosing back problems.

Keep in mind that your doctor probably won't use all of these tests. In fact, he may not use any of them. Your doctor may use a different method, based on your symptoms or other findings.

Also, keep in mind that even a high-tech test doesn't always provide clues to a diagnosis. In most cases of back pain, a precise cause may never be found. But that doesn't mean that you and your doctor won't find an effective treatment for your pain – don't give up hope! These tests will help your doctor narrow down the possibilities so the right treatments can be identified.

Imaging Tests

Imaging tests are those that use radiation or magnetic force to take pictures of the inside of the body and thus may be used to diagnose the cause of back pain.

It's important to note, however, that just because an imaging test shows a problem, the problem isn't necessarily the source of pain. For example, a large percentage of older people have osteoarthritic changes, disc bulges and even herniated discs in the spine that can be seen by X-ray, yet only a small percentage of those people have back pain. Thus, if you are having back pain and an X-ray shows OA or a bulging or herniated disc, these might be the source of your pain – or they might not. That's why it's important to evaluate the findings of imaging tests (in fact, any test) in the context of a medical history and physical exam.

X-rays

The oldest and most widely used imaging test is the plain X-ray. To take an X-ray, a technician will have you lie on a table while an X-ray machine passes low-level radiation through your body to project a picture called a radiograph on a piece of film. Your doctor may recommend an X-ray if he suspects osteoarthritis, a vertebral fracture or an alignment problem with your spine. X-rays also show certain bony changes in the spine, helping doctors diagnose such diseases as ankylosing spondylitis and the other spondyloarthropathies.

A plain X-ray will show only the bones and spaces between the bones where your discs are. If a soft-tissue problem is suspected, a different test will be necessary.

While the X-ray itself is not painful, some people with back problems may find it difficult to lie down or get into the right position for the test. If you anticipate problems or have difficulty during an X-ray, it's important to let the technician know. He or she may be able to help.

Because of the low levels of radiation used, X-rays are safe. If you are pregnant (a potential cause of back pain) or suspect you are pregnant, you should not have an X-ray. In addition, if you are a man and there is a possibility that you will later want to have children, the technician may cover your reproductive organs with a lead shield. Unfortunately, it is impossible to shield a woman's reproductive organs and still get an X-ray of the lower spine, so if you are a woman and think there is any chance you might be pregnant, don't hesitate to let the technician know – speak up!

Computerized Tomography (CT or CAT) Scan

Often referred to as **CT scans** or CAT scans, computerized tomography involves using a computer to record two-dimensional "slice" images of your body and, in some cases, turning those slices into a three-dimensional view of the back. This procedure can help your doctor see if there is a ruptured or degenerated disc, spinal stenosis, tumors or infections of the spinal cord. The CT scan shows structures of the spine that a plain X-ray can't. It also uses more radiation than a traditional X-ray, but the amount used is safe.

To perform a CT scan, the technician will have you lie on your back on a narrow table, which will then be inserted into a cylinder-shaped machine. The scan itself is painless; however, doctors sometimes inject a contrast agent into a vein to illuminate the structures of your spine on the scan, and some people find the injection painful. Also, some people may find it difficult to lie still on their back for the duration of the procedure, which is generally between 30 and 45 minutes.

Magnetic Resonance Imaging (MRI)

Magnetic Resonance Imaging (MRI) is a procedure in which a very strong magnet is used to pass a force through the body to create a clear, detailed image of a cross section of the body. It is harmless and does not expose the body to radiation.

The advantage of MRI scans over plain X-rays and CT scans is that MRI provides clear, detailed images of soft-tissue structures, such as the muscles, cartilage, ligaments, discs, tendons and blood vessels, in addition to the bones. When diagnosing back pain, this capability can be an important advantage, as back pain is more likely to be related to soft-tissue problems than to problems with the bones.

An MRI is appropriate for diagnosing tumors and infections of the spine. It is the best test for detecting whether there is pressure on a nerve or on the spinal cord. It may also be used for early diagnosis of a form of arthritis affecting the spine, such as ankylosing spondylitis or rheumatoid arthritis.

To perform an MRI, the technician will have you lie on a narrow scanning table that is then inserted into a narrow magnetic tunnel. The procedure is safe and physically painless, although some people find it difficult to lie still inside the machine for the 45 to 60 minutes required to perform the test.

If your doctor orders an MRI, let him or her know if you have any metal in your body, such as a prosthetic joint, surgical clip or shrapnel. If you are claustrophobic, you can ask about the possibility of having an open MRI. Be aware, however, that the majority of open MRI machines don't provide the same resolution and quality of images that closed machines do.

Bone Scan

In a bone scan, a small amount of radioactive dye is injected into a vein in your arm and allowed to circulate through your body, including the bones of your spine, for a couple of hours.

A special camera is then used to scan the area in question and produce a picture. The scan works by detecting any area of the spine that has an increase in blood flow and bone-forming cell activity, which could possibly indicate a tumor, infection or fracture.

Discogram

A **discogram** is a test used to view and assess the internal structure of a disc and to determine if the disc is a source of pain. To perform a discogram, a doctor injects a radiopaque dye (a dye that shows up on radiological scans) into the disc or discs being examined. The doctor then performs a CT scan, in which any tears, scars or changes in the disc are illuminated. If a damaged disc has been a source of pain, injecting the dye should help you and your doctor identify the problematic disc by recreating the type of pain you've been experiencing.

Unlike other imaging tests, discograms are invasive (meaning they involve entering the body) and for that reason they have the potential for complications, such as infection. Discograms typically are performed on people who are scheduled for surgery. By locating the precise source of pain, they can help the doctor plan appropriate surgery.

Dual Energy X-ray Absorptiometry (DEXA or DXA)

Although it is not used to diagnose the cause of back pain, **DEXA** is used to diagnose osteoporosis, the cause of most vertebral fractures, which can be painful. DEXA uses a small amount of radiation to determine the density, or thickness, of bone in the spine and other areas of the body.

If osteoporosis is detected, your doctor can recommend treatment – including medication (see "Osteoporosis Medications" in Chapter 3), diet and exercise – to help prevent future fractures. Although DEXA is one of the most widely used tests for bone density, there are several others, including:

- Peripheral dual energy X-ray absorptiometry (pDXA)
- Single X-ray absorptiometry (SXA)
- Quantitative ultrasound (QUS)
- Quantitative computed tomography (QCT)
- Peripheral quantitative computed tomography (pQCT)
- Radiographic absorptiometry (RA)

Nerve Tests

Nerve tests, also called electrodiagnostic studies, are used to determine whether the electrical activity of nerves has been disrupted as a result of problems in the back. The most common electrodiagnostic test used in back pain is electromyography.

Symptoms of Back Problems

Although you should always see a physician to confirm a diagnosis of potentially serious or lingering back problems, your symptoms could give you some clues as to the source of your pain. Following are just a few of the more common causes of back problems and their specific symptoms.

Symptom	Possible or likely cause(s)
Sudden, jabbing pain when bending or lifting, accompanied by a temporary inability to stand upright	Muscle strain or spasm, degenerative disc disease, facet syndrome
Pain that is sharp, debilitating and travels down one leg	Herniated disc
Sore lower back accompanied by chronic fatigue and muscle pain in other areas; poor sleep	Fibromyalgia

Symptom	Possible or likely cause(s)
Pain in the spine that is worse after prolonged sitting or inactivity, particularly if accompanied by a decreased ability to twist, bend or turn, or by inflammation in joints, such as the shoulders, ankles and knees	Ankylosing spondylitis
Pain in the lower spine, stiffness that lasts for about 30 minutes after getting up in the morning, possibly limited motion of the spine	Osteoarthritis
Severe, sudden pain localized to a specific site of the back	Fractured vertebra
Pain in the buttock, leg or thigh when standing or walking; numbness, weakness and tingling in legs	Spinal stenosis
Pain felt deep inside the back that doesn't correlate with rest or activity	Constipation, menstrual cramps, endometriosis, bowel inflammation

Electromyography

Electromyography (also called EMG or myogram) is a procedure that involves inserting needle electrodes through the skin into a muscle. The electrical activity detected by the electrodes is displayed on a piece of equipment called an oscilloscope that resembles a TV screen with wavy lines crossing it.

The presence, size and shape of the waves produced on the screen tell your doctor how able your muscle is to respond to nerve stimulation, and can assist in the diagnosis of problems involving the nervous system.

People undergoing electromyography may experience mild to moderate pain from the procedure. If you undergo the procedure, plan to rest a while afterward and take acetaminophen for pain, if necessary. (Be sure to check with your doctor if you are already taking pain medication for your back problem.) If acetaminophen doesn't relieve your pain, you may want to ask your doctor about a stronger pain medication to take for a brief time after the procedure.

Electromyography is most useful for determining whether problems with the spinal nerve roots are the cause of pain in the legs, and if so, which nerve roots are involved. It is not particularly useful for back pain alone.

Blood tests

Generally, blood work is not part of the work-up for back pain; however, in some cases, the results of certain blood tests can assist the diagnostic process by helping doctors differentiate mechanical from medical causes of pain. Such tests include:

Complete blood count (CBC) – a test performed on the blood that shows the levels of the different types of blood cells. Changes in blood cell levels could indicate such problems as infection or an inflammatory disease, such as rheumatoid arthritis or ankylosing spondylitis.

Erythrocyte sedimentation rate (ESR or "sed rate") – a blood test used to detect and measure inflammation. The higher the sed rate, the more inflammation is present. A high sed rate could indicate a number of possibilities, including an inflammatory disease, infection or, in rare cases, a tumor.

Tissue Typing – The finding of a specific genetic marker called HLA-B27 in the blood can help a doctor identify a possible diagnosis of ankylosing spondylitis (a form of arthritis that primarily affects the spine and sacroiliac joints) or reactive arthritis (a similar disease characterized by inflammation of the joints, eyes and urethra). Although the genetic marker is more common in people with these diseases, perfectly healthy people can have it. For that reason, a positive HLA-B27 test alone does not mean you have one of these diseases.

Psychological Tests

Although psychological stresses are rarely the sole cause of back pain, they can certainly contribute to it or result from it. For that reason, some doctors may recommend their patients undergo psychological testing, often along with one or more of the medical tests described previously.

In a psychological test, a professional (such as a psychologist or psychiatrist) who is trained to help people with pain problems will interview you about such issues as your family life, work situation, medication or alcohol use or abuse, pain history and any litigation or compensation related to your pain.

The professional will also ask questions to help assess your mood, energy level and ability to sleep and concentrate.

The Fibromyalgia Exam

Many of the conditions that cause back pain cannot be diagnosed through X-rays, blood tests or even the most technologically sophisticated imaging tests available. Yet one condition, fibromyalgia syndrome, can be diagnosed only through a medical history and physical exam.

One of the key determinants of a fibromyalgia diagnosis is the presence of tender points, or tender, painful areas in the muscles, tendons or places where the bone can be felt through the skin. Many people with fibromyalgia don't even realize they have tender points until the physician applies pressure to these points during the exam.

The location of these tender points is fairly consistent from person to person. There are 18 recognized tender points in fibromyalgia. In general, to receive a fibromyalgia diagnosis, you must have at least 11 tender points, in combination with widespread pain.

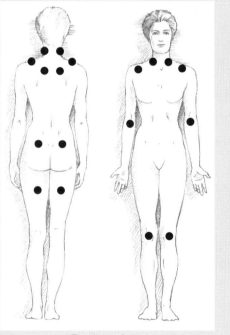

Tender points:
Areas where fibromyalgia pain may occur

The results of psychological testing can help your doctor better understand your pain and, with that understanding, develop a treatment approach that includes some stress management techniques, which we will discuss in Chapter 9.

Working With Your Doctor: Finding the Right Fit

Although most cases of back pain come and go with little treatment, back pain can be a long-term problem with many potential causes and just as many – or more – possible solutions. When back pain lingers, managing it may require a team effort involving you, your doctor and other health-care providers.

While the best doctor-patient situation is one in which there is some give-and-take, perhaps what's most important is that you see eye to eye with your doctor. Problems arise when there is a discrepancy between the ways you and your doctor prefer to work. If you want to take a role in your health care, but your doctor expects you to follow orders without question, it may be time to find a new doctor.

Before you do that, make sure you're not asking or expecting too much of your doctor. While your doctor should be willing to answer questions and be open to the possibility of different treatments you would like to try, no doctor has the time to answer endless lists of queries from every patient.

A doctor who merely agrees with everything you suggest is not good for you either. And prescribing – or even condoning – every treatment you mention can be downright dangerous!

You'll be working as a team with your doctor and/or other health-care professionals you select, and your goal will be to find the best treatments for your back pain. There are a number of options, including drugs, exercise, massage, water therapy and, if necessary, surgical treatments.

In the following chapters, we will discuss some of the many treatment options that are available to you. Finding the treatment or treatments that work for your situation may be fairly simple or it could be a long task requiring trial and error. Together, you and your health-care team will find the right methods for your situation.

chapter 3:

Treating Pain With Medications

When you experience the initial twinges of back pain, your inclination may be to pop a couple of aspirin tablets or one of the similar over-the-counter pain relievers. For many people, over-the-counter medications taken for a few days are sufficient to relieve minor back pain, while more persistent or severe pain may require stronger medication available only with a doctor's prescription.

In this chapter, we'll take a look at some of the most common medication options for back pain. We'll also answer some common questions about medications and offer some useful tips on using them wisely. As you read, however, keep in mind that medications aren't the only route to relief. Nor are they always the best or safest treatment for your pain.

Some back pain responds sufficiently to conservative non-medication measures alone, while other cases may require more invasive treatments, including surgery. In all cases, medication – if used – should be part of a well-rounded treatment plan that includes rest, exercise, non-medication therapies, healthy lifestyle habits, stress reduction and, if necessary, surgery.

In this chapter, we focus only on medications that are taken by mouth (oral), injected or rubbed on (topical) for relief. We'll answer some commonly asked questions about medications and discuss the specific medications that are used for back pain and some of the various conditions that cause such pain.

In the next three chapters, we'll look at some of the other many methods for relieving back pain and – if all goes well – preventing its return.

Prescription vs. OTC: What's the Difference?

You're scanning the shelves of your local pharmacy for something to ease your aching back, and you find literally dozens of medications labeled with words like pain reliever, non-aspirin pain reliever, backache pills or nighttime pain reliever. What is the difference between all of these medications, and how do they differ from the medications a doctor prescribes?

Essentially the difference between these and prescription medications is that you don't need a doctor's written order – or phone call to the pharmacy – to get them. But they are still serious medicine.

When it comes to pain-relieving medications that may be useful for treating your back pain, the ones you'll find over the counter are the analgesic medication acetaminophen (*Tylenol*); and five nonsteroidal anti-inflammatory drugs (NSAIDs), ibuprofen (*Advil, Motrin*), naproxen sodium (*Aleve*), ketoprofen (*Orudis KT*), aspirin (*Bayer, Bufferin*) and magnesium salicylate (*Bayer Select* and *Doan's Pills*). Aspirin and magnesium salicylate are a subset of NSAIDs referred to as *salicylates*, meaning they contain salicylic acid, the active ingredient found in aspirin.

Although these drugs come in many formulations and in combinations with other ingredients (such as caffeine to speed pain relief, antihistamines to cause drowsiness or a diuretic to ease bloating) these are the only over-the-counter medications taken orally that ease pain.

Increasingly, drugs that were once available only by prescription are becoming available over the counter. Between 1984 and 1994, about one drug per year switched from prescription-only to over-the-counter status. In 1996 alone, 13 prescription-only drugs became available over the counter.

The increasing availability of medications without a doctor's prescription has benefits and drawbacks. On the positive side, getting a medication has never been more convenient and less expensive. You don't need an appointment with a physician if all you need is something to ease the pain of a muscle strain.

On the negative side, people are more likely than ever to self-medicate, not realizing they have a condition that requires the care of a physician. People also tend to think that anything they get over the counter is safe and that they can adjust the dosage as they see fit. This is not true. Even if you are taking an over-the-counter medication, it's important to follow the directions exactly. You should contact your doctor promptly if you suspect an adverse reaction or if symptoms don't improve.

It's also important to understand that over-the-counter medications may be similar or identical to the ones prescribed by your doctor. Therefore, taking an over-the-counter medication along with your prescription may lead to an overdose. Tell your doctor about all the medications you are taking at any time for your back pain, including over-the-counter medicines.

Generic vs. Brand-Name: What's the Difference?

At some point when you're filling a prescription, the pharmacist may ask you, "Do you want the generic?" How should you answer? A *generic* version of a drug contains the same helpful medicine as the *brand-name* version of a drug. Is a generic as good as the brand-name medication? What's the difference?

As far as you're concerned, the only difference will probably be the cost. Choosing generics is likely to cost you significantly less than buying the brand-name counterpart – like the difference between the store-brand green beans and the brand-name variety. Aside from the product's packaging and the perhaps minor differences in taste and appearance, you are getting essentially the same vegetable – or medicine.

Here's why: When a company develops a new drug, it applies for a patent, which prohibits anyone else from marketing the drug for 20 years. This time of exclusivity allows the company to recoup the costs of developing and testing the drug, which averages about $360 million per medication. After the patent has expired, other manufacturers may duplicate and market their own versions of the drug, called generics. Because makers of generic drugs don't have to repeat the extensive clinical trials to prove the safety and efficacy of their drugs, their expenses are much less, and they can pass those savings along to you.

Even though generic manufacturers don't have to repeat the same rigorous tests that the manufacturer of the original drug must pass, there are certain requirements for companies that manufacture generics. Foremost, they have to prove that their drug is chemically identical to the brand-name version – that is, its active ingredient, the ingredient that addresses the pain, inflammation or other physical problem, is the same. However, the inert ingredients, such as dyes and fillers, may be different. If you are allergic to certain dyes or fillers, such as corn, that could be an important difference between generic and brand-name medications.

In the vast majority of cases, you'll probably never know the difference between a brand-name and generic drug. In the rare event that you don't get the same relief as you do from the brand-name medication or that you experience a reaction to a nonactive ingredient in a particular medication, your best bet is to try the same medication from another manufacturer. Ask your doctor or pharmacist for a recommendation.

Medications for Back Pain

Treating back pain may require medications purely for pain relief, medications to treat the cause of pain or some combination of the two. Following are some of the types of medications that may be part of your treatment regimen.

ANALGESICS

Many people with back pain benefit from analgesic, or pain-relieving, medications. Analgesic medications are used purely for pain relief – that is, they don't work against inflammation the way nonsteroidal anti-inflammatory drugs do. (See the discussion of NSAIDs later in this chapter.) Analgesics can be taken orally or applied topically.

The most commonly used and readily available oral analgesic is acetaminophen (*Tylenol*). For many people, acetaminophen alone may be sufficient to ease back pain. Acetaminophen can be purchased over the counter under a variety of different trade and store names and is often the active ingredient in products labeled "aspirin-free pain reliever."

For more severe pain or the acute pain of a vertebral fracture or back surgery, doctors often prescribe narcotic analgesics such as codeine, oxycodone (*OxyContin, Roxicodone*), propoxyphene hydrochloride (*Darvon, PP-Cap*) or tramadol (*Ultram*).

Narcotic analgesics carry side effects, including drowsiness, grogginess, constipation and the potential for dependence. For that reason, doctors may prescribe them for acute back pain, but hesitate to prescribe them for an ongoing pain condition. Acetaminophen, on the other hand, is rarely associated with side effects if taken as directed. It is one of the most commonly prescribed and used medications for back pain.

Some medications combine acetaminophen with a narcotic for added pain relief. Such drugs include acetaminophen with codeine (*Fioricet, Phenaphen* with *Codeine, Tylenol* with *Codeine*), hydrocodone with acetaminophen (*Dolacet, Hydrocet, Lorcet, Lortab, Vicodin*) and tramadol with acetaminophen (*Ultracet*).

Topical Analgesics

If you find you can't take oral analgesics or if oral analgesics don't completely relieve pain in the soft tissues of your back, you may want to try one of the many analgesic salves, creams, rubs and balms available over the counter. While these products usually are used on peripheral (away from the center of the body) joints, such as the knees or joints of the hands, you might find them useful – and safe – for back pain.

Unlike most other pain-relieving medications, which are swallowed or injected, these rubs work only on the area into which you rub them, minimizing the risk of systemic side effects.

The effects of topical analgesics come from one or more of a variety of active ingredients. Here are some of the most common ones:

Capsaicin – A highly purified natural ingredient found in cayenne peppers, capsaicin works by depleting the amount of a neurotransmitter called substance P that is believed to send pain messages to the brain. For the first couple of weeks of use, the ingredient may cause burning or stinging. Capsaicin is available under the product names *Arthoflex Max-Cap, Zostrix, Capzasin-P* and others. *Menthacin* is a topical cream that includes both capsaicin and counterirritants.

Counterirritants – Like stepping on your toe to take your mind off a headache, counterirritants stimulate or irritate the nerve endings to distract the brain's attention from musculoskeletal pain. Counterirritants encompass such substances as menthol, oil of wintergreen, camphor, eucalyptus oil, turpentine oil, dihydrochloride and methylnicotinate and are found in such products as *ArthriCare, Eucalyptamint, Icy Hot* and *Therapeutic Mineral Ice*.

Salicylates – Like the salicylates found in many oral pain relievers, these compounds may work by inhibiting prostaglandins. Topically, they work primarily as counterirritants, stimulating or irritating nerve endings. Brand-name examples of topical analgesics containing salicylates include *Aspercreme, Ben-Gay, Flexall, Mobisyl* and *Sportscreme*.

A NOTE FOR YOUR NOSE: If you've ever used a topical analgesic, you know that they can be smelly. The very substances used to stimulate or irritate your nerve endings may irritate your sense of smell! For that reason, topical analgesics may not be an appropriate choice for pain relief if you are on your way to a business meeting or a friend's wedding. Before using a topical analgesic when you'll be out and among people, take a whiff and see if it's objectionable. When selecting a topical cream in the drugstore, your pharmacist may be able to suggest some less smelly products.

NONSTEROIDAL ANTI-INFLAMMATORY DRUGS

The class of drugs called NSAIDs includes one of the oldest and most widely used medications – aspirin – as well as the popular over-the-counter medications ibuprofen (*Advil, Motrin IB, Nuprin*), ketoprofen (*Actron, Orudis KT*) and naproxen sodium (*Aleve*), which are available in higher doses by prescription. Nearly two dozen other NSAIDs are available by prescription under various generic and brand names. (See "Generic vs. Brand Name: What's the Difference?" on page 43.)

All NSAIDs ease pain and inflammation by blocking the production of bodily chemicals called *prostaglandins*, which also play a role in numerous other bodily functions, including blood clotting, kidney function and stomach lining protection.

While NSAIDs are an important component of a back-pain treatment plan for many people, they are not without risks. The most common side effects of NSAIDs are related to the gastrointestinal system and include stomach or abdominal pain, nausea, indigestion, heartburn and vomiting. (To learn how you and your doctor can ease such problems, see "Gut Relief: Easing NSAIDs' Unwanted Effects," on page 49.) People who take high doses of NSAIDs or take them long-term for a chronic condition also face a risk of gastric ulcers with bleeding.

If you are at increased risk for ulcers (see "Risk Factor for Ulcers," on page 48) and need NSAIDs to relieve pain and inflammation, speak to your doctor about the advisability of taking one of the newer classes of NSAIDs called COX-2 inhibitors. The drugs, which include celecoxib (*Celebrex*), rofecoxib (*Vioxx*) and valdecoxib (*Bextra*), have many of the benefits of traditional NSAIDs, but with less risk of gastric ulcers.

AN IMPORTANT NOTE: As with any drugs, these newer NSAIDs aren't for everyone. At least one study suggested taking a COX-2 inhibitor could slightly increase your risk of a heart attack. If you have heart disease risk factors, let your doctor know before starting one of these drugs. He or she may recommend taking low-dose aspirin (60 milligrams to 80 milligrams daily) along with the drug to help reduce your risk of a heart attack.

Risk Factors for Ulcers

You may be at increased risk for a gastric ulcer if you:

- Are over age 65
- Have had stomach ulcers in the past
- Consume more than three alcoholic drinks daily
- Use blood-thinning medications
- Have a bacterial infection called *Helicobacter pylori*
- Use glucocorticoid medications, such as prednisone

Gut Relief: Easing NSAIDs' Unwanted Effects

If you take nonsteroidal anti-inflammatory drugs (NSAIDs) frequently or long-term for chronic pain, there's a good chance you'll experience some stomach upset or heartburn with them – at least from time to time. For some people taking NSAIDs, gastrointestinal (GI) problems are frequent and sometimes severe. The most severe is the development of gastric (stomach) ulcers and the complication of bleeding or obstruction of the bowel.

The only sure way to prevent gastric ulcers and other NSAID side effects is to stop taking NSAIDs. Aside from that painful prospect, there are several methods the doctor can recommend to significantly reduce NSAIDs' GI risks.

- NEWER, GENTLER DRUGS. If stomach ulcers are a problem, a relatively new class of NSAIDs called cyclooxygenase-2 (COX-2) inhibitors can provide the relief that traditional NSAIDs do, but with a much-reduced ulcer risk. The COX-2 drugs include celecoxib (*Celebrex*), rofecoxib (*Vioxx*), valdecoxib (*Bextra*) and several other drugs still in development and clinical testing. In addition, switching from a traditional NSAID to a COX-2 drug may ease other GI problems associated with NSAIDs (including stomach pain, nausea, heartburn or indigestion).

- STOMACH PROTECTION. If you've had stomach ulcers in the past or are at high risk for them, your doctor may prescribe a medication called misoprostol (*Cytotec*) along with your regular NSAID.

continued p. 50

continued from p. 49

Misoprostol is a synthetic prostaglandin that replaces the stomach-protecting substances that traditional NSAIDs wipe out.

- ACID RELIEF. When NSAIDs cause stomach upset or indigestion, doctors often prescribe or recommend drugs that reduce the body's production of gastric acid. Two such categories of medication are:
    - **Histamine blockers (H2 blockers)**, which include cimetidine (*Tagamet*), ranitidine hydrochloride (*Zantac*), famotidine (*Pepcid*) and nizatidine (*Axid Pulvules*).
    - **Proton pump inhibitors**, which include omeprazole (*Prilosec)*, lansoprazole (*Prevacid*) and esomeprazole magnesium (*Nexium*).

Although many of these drugs are available over the counter, you should always check with your doctor before using one along with an NSAID. The reason: By relieving stomach symptoms, these drugs could potentially mask problems requiring medical evaluation.

- MEDICATION COMBO. If you don't like the idea of taking another drug along with your NSAIDs, one manufacturer has combined the NSAID diclofenac sodium and misoprostol in a single product. The drug, called *Arthrotec*, is available only by prescription.

STEROIDS

When inflammation within the spinal column causes nerve-root irritation and swelling, doctors sometimes administer a potent anti-inflammatory medication to reduce inflammation and ease pain.

Steroids are typically injected directly into the epidural space – the area between the dura mater (the outer membrane of the spinal cord) and the vertebrae – to deliver medication directly to the site of inflammation. (To learn more about steroid injections and other types of injection therapy, see Chapter 4: "Injection and Implant Procedures.")

ANTIDEPRESSANTS, MUSCLE RELAXANTS AND SIMILAR DRUGS

Antidepressants

Doctors often prescribe tricyclic antidepressants, such as amitriptyline (*Elavil*) and nortriptyline (*Pamelor*) for chronic low back pain. To break the pain cycle, doctors often prescribe antidepressant drugs at doses lower than those used to treat depression. At larger doses, the drugs can reduce pain and ease depression, which can result from and contribute to back pain. Antidepressants may cause drowsiness, which can be helpful if back pain makes it difficult to sleep.

Muscle Relaxants

Muscle relaxants may be used to ease muscle spasms. For pain relief, they are often prescribed along with NSAIDs. Commonly prescribed muscle relaxants include cyclobenzaprine (*Flexeril*), orphenadrine (*Norflex*) and carisoprodol (*Soma*). Like antidepressants, muscle relaxants may cause drowsiness, so they can be helpful if back pain keeps you awake at night.

Similar Drugs

Two other drugs used to treat pain and muscle spasms associated with back pain are:

Gabapentin (*Neurotonin*) – A medication that has proven useful for many types of neurological pain, gabapentin may be helpful when nerve-root irritation causes back pain. Gabapentin may cause mild drowsiness.

Tizanidine (*Zanaflex*) – Tizanadine works on the central nervous system to relax the muscles. It is particularly helpful for chronic musculoskeletal pain. By easing muscle spasms, tizanidine makes it easier – or at least possible – to do rehabilitative exercises. (For more about rehabilitation and exercise for back pain, see 108.)

ARTHRITIS MEDICATIONS

The same NSAIDs widely used for other causes of back pain are also used to ease the pain and inflammation of arthritis. However, if back pain, stiffness or damage is caused by an inflammatory disease process, such as ankylosing spondylitis or reactive arthritis, getting the pain under control will also require getting the disease under control. Doctors prescribe two types of drugs to control the disease process – disease-modifying antirheumatic drugs (DMARDs) and biologic response modifiers. Following is a brief description of both types.

DMARDs

Disease-modifying antirheumatic drugs (DMARDs) are a class of medications doctors may prescribe for ankylosing spondylitis, as well as
some other inflammatory forms of arthritis that may affect the back. As
the name suggests, DMARDs actually modify the course of disease,
slowing or perhaps even stopping its progression. Most of these drugs
work by suppressing the immune system, which is involved in the joint
damage that occurs in ankylosing spondylitis and other diseases.

If your doctor prescribes a disease-modifying antirheumatic drug,
don't expect quick results, as these drugs often take several weeks or
even months to produce effects. Most people will find the results well
worth the wait.

The following medications fall into the DMARD category: methotrex-
ate, leflunomide (*Arava*), sulfasalazine (*Azulfidine*) and hydroxychloroquine sulfate (*Plaquenil*).

Biologic Response Modifiers

Unlike traditional DMARDs, which may cause widespread suppression
of the immune system, biologic response modifiers (BRMs, or
biologic agents) target specific immune system components,
such as chemical messengers called cytokines, which play a
role in the inflammation and damage of the disease.

Etanercept (*Enbrel*) and infliximab (*Remicade*) work by different chemical actions to block an inflammatory cytokine called
tumor necrosis factor (TNF), which is believed to play a role in anky-

losing spondylitis and some other diseases. As a result, these agents retard the inflammatory response and ease the signs and symptoms of ankylosing spondylitis.

While some doctors reserve biologic agents for patients whose arthritis hasn't responded well to more conventional therapies, others are starting to prescribe them earlier in the disease process in an effort to ward off or reduce permanent joint damage.

Etanercept is administered by an injection beneath the skin. Infliximab is given by intravenous infusion.

OSTEOPOROSIS MEDICATIONS

While osteoporosis itself isn't painful, the fractures that can result from osteoporosis are. Medications such as analgesics and NSAIDs may be used to control the pain from fractures, yet it's equally important – if not more so – to treat the underlying bone disease.

Three categories of medications are used to promote bone growth or suppress bone loss. Doctors prescribe these medications to prevent fractures. The specific medication your doctor prescribes will depend on a number of factors, including your sex, medical history, and your and your doctor's preference.

Hormones

Hormones that naturally occur in the body help regulate the balance of bone breakdown and regrowth. When certain hormones are deficient, bone can break down faster than it is replaced, resulting in thin, fragile bones. Administering hormonal medications, however, can help tip the breakdown/regrowth balance in your bones' favor.

There are two types of hormonal medications for osteoporosis:

Estrogen – Still the most widely used osteoporosis medication for post-menopausal women is the female hormone estrogen (*Premarin, Estratab, Menest*). Prior to menopause, high levels of estrogen in the body help to keep bone strong by causing the death of cells that are responsible for bone degradation. For women who have not had a hysterectomy, doctors prescribe estrogen in combination with the hormone progesterone (*Premphase, Prempro*) to minimize any adverse effects of estrogen on the uterus. If you are going through menopause and experiencing troublesome hot flashes and other symptoms, estrogen replacement can ease those symptoms as well as bone loss.

Calcitonin – If you've suffered a vertebral fracture, another hormonal drug, calcitonin, may offer some pain-relieving effects while helping to prevent future fractures. Calcitonin is similar to a hormone produced by our parathyroid glands (two pairs of endocrine glands that are situated behind or within the thyroid gland). Naturally occurring in the body, parathyroid hormone controls the distribution of calcium and phosphate in the body and has been shown to have an effect on bone growth. Calcitonin can be administered by injection (*Calcimar, Miacalcin*) or nasal spray (*Miacalcin*). (*Miacalcin* is available as both an injection and nasal spray.)

Bisphosphonates

A class of medication used in the treatment of bone diseases, including Paget's disease, bisphosphonates are being used increasingly in the treatment of osteoporosis as well, because they inhibit bone breakdown. In recent years, two bisphosphonate medications, alendronate (*Fosamax*) and risedronate sodium (*Actonel*), were approved for osteoporosis. Risedronate sodium is approved specifically for glucocorticoid-induced osteoporosis. Unlike many of the other medications used for osteoporosis, bisphosphonates are appropriate for men.

Selective estrogen receptor molecules

One of the newest classes of medications for osteoporosis, selective estrogen receptor molecules (SERMs), including raloxifene hydrochloride (*Evista*), work much like estrogen to slow bone loss. The major advantage is that they lack some of estrogen's side effects, mainly those related to breast and uterine tissue, making them an attractive alternative to estrogen replacement for women at increased risk of breast or uterine cancer.

OTHER DRUGS

Widely different medical treatments may be prescribed, depending on the source of your back pain. For example, the treatment for a tumor of the spine would be different from treatment for a bladder infection or endometriosis. Specific drug treatments for all of the various and uncommon causes of pain are beyond the scope of this book. However, with a proper diagnosis, your primary care doctor or a specialist, if necessary, can prescribe the appropriate medical treatment for your specific problem.

Understanding Medications: Where To Learn More

Because of the variety of medications used for back problems and the emergence of new medications, keeping up with your medications, what they're supposed to do and how to take them can be difficult. When you have a question about your medication, it's always best to consult your doctor or pharmacist. The following resources also provide information to help you better understand the medications you take.

BOOKS

United States Pharmacopoeia Dispensing Information (USP DI) Volume II Advice for the Patient, Drug Information in Lay Language (2001, Micromedex, $75). Offers easy-to-understand information on more than 11,000 brand name and generic medications marketed in the United States and Canada. To order, call 800/877-6209 or visit the Micromedex Web site at www.micromedex.com/products.

Physician's Desk Reference (PDR) (2001, Medical Economics, $77.95). Features up-to-date FDA-approved information on more than 4,000 prescription drugs and photos of the most prescribed drugs. To order, call 800/232-7379 or visit the Medical Economics Web site at www.medec.com/html/products.

PDR for Nonprescription Drugs and Dietary Supplements (2001, Medical Economics, $48.95). Contains detailed descriptions of the most commonly used nonprescription drugs and preparations, along with full-color photographs of hundreds of over-the-counter drugs for quick identification. To order, call 800/232-7379 or visit the Medical Economics Web site at www.medec.com/html/products.

WEB SITES

www.OnHealth.com/conditions/resources/pharmacy/index.asp offers clear information on thousands of prescription and over-the-counter medications, listed by generic and brand name. Also features a tool that allows you to check for drugs that interact with one another.

www.safemedication.com, a Web site of the American Health-System Pharmacists, offers important information on using medications safely and wisely.

www.FDA.gov, the Web site of the Food and Drug Administration, offers a search engine for looking up information about medications and numerous food- and drug-related subjects.

OTHERS

The Arthritis Foundation. The Arthritis Foundation magazine, *Arthritis Today*, publishes an annual guide to drugs used in the treatment of arthritis and related conditions. The Arthritis Foundation offers brochures and other resources on medications used in arthritis and related conditions, including back pain. To inquire about a specific brochure or to order a free copy of *Arthritis Today's Drug Guide*, contact your local Arthritis Foundation office or call 800/283-7800. You can also search the Arthritis Foundation Web site for general information at www.arthritis.org.

Pharmacy handouts. Most pharmacies include a printout with each prescription, telling you how to take the medication, and informing you of possible side effects and what to do if you experience them. Read and become familiar with the printout before starting your course of medication, and be sure to discuss any concerns with your doctor or pharmacist.

Package labels and inserts. Each medication, over-the-counter or prescription, comes from the manufacturer with a package insert detailing how the medication should be taken, who should and shouldn't take it, how it works and the side effects associated with it. Inserts can be found in over-the-counter medication packages. For most prescription medications, you will never see the package insert unless you ask for it.

Beyond Medication

While medications can ease back pain and, in some cases, modify or stop an underlying disease that leads to pain, medication is most effective when used in conjunction with a well-rounded treatment plan. In the following chapters, we'll discuss some of the many ways other than medication to treat back pain.

Questions To Ask About Medications

To get the greatest benefit – and least risk of adverse effects – from your medications, it's important to know as much as possible about what your doctor is prescribing. Here are some questions you might want to ask your doctor or pharmacist:

- What is the name of the medication?
- How long has it been on the market?
- How is this medication expected to help me?
- Are there any special instructions for taking this drug?
- Is it habit-forming?
- Are there side effects I should be aware of?
- What should I do if I experience side effects?
- How long should I expect to wait before noticing effects?
- What should I do if I miss a dose of this medication?
- Is a generic version of the drug available?
- Will my insurance cover this medication?
- If the medication is expensive, is there something similar that is less expensive?
- Is there anything else I should know about this medication?

chapter 4

Injection and Implant Procedures

There are many different treatments for back pain. Taking lots of drugs (which many people find unpleasant) or undergoing surgery are not your only options. Plenty of medical options that fall between medications and surgery may be very effective treatments for your back pain. Among those options are **injections** and **implants**, procedures that you can discuss with your doctor. Let's look at these potentially helpful therapies now.

Injections are procedures that involve using a needle to deliver a stimulus, medication or other substance directly to the source of back pain or damage. Implant therapies are those that work through a pain-relieving device placed surgically inside the body. The devices work by delivering either a medication or stimulus to the spine.

While some of these therapies have been used for decades, some are relatively new and just starting to gain acceptance. Others are controversial, with little scientific evidence to support their use.

In general, injections are used for people with chronic pain that has not responded to other therapies. The success of injections varies and depends largely on the problem that's causing pain, the correct placement of the needle and the experience of the doctor giving the injection.

Most often, implants are used to treat people who have had back surgery, but have found that surgery didn't relieve their pain sufficiently. When back surgery to correct the cause of a person's pain doesn't provide relief, we say the person has "failed back syndrome." Implants or injections may offer these people relief for their debilitating pain.

In this chapter, we'll discuss the most common injections and implantable therapies used for back pain.

Injections

Several different types of doctors may perform injections, including orthopaedic surgeons, anesthesiologists, physiatrists, rheumatologists and radiologists. The amount of pain people feel with injections is highly variable. Some people report moderate pain with injections; others say they experience virtually no pain at all. Even if injections do cause some pain, most people would prefer them to invasive surgery. Usually an anesthetic (pain-killing medication) is administered with the injection, helping to ease any pain associated with the procedure.

The risks associated with injections are variable, too, and include infection, bleeding, nerve damage or a puncture of the dura mater (known as a "wet tap"), the outer membrane of the spinal cord, which can cause a headache for up to a few days afterwards. Fortunately, all of these risks are rare and when they do occur, they usually are not serious or long-lasting.

Injections are safe for most people and are performed on an outpatient basis. If you have a procedure in the morning, in most cases, you'll be home that afternoon.

There are numerous types of injections. The best one for you, should you need one, will depend on your particular problem.

EPIDURAL STEROID INJECTION

When inflammation within the spinal column causes nerve-root irritation and swelling, doctors sometimes administer a potent anti-inflammatory medication to reduce inflammation and ease pain.

Steroids typically are injected directly into the epidural space – the area between the dura mater and the vertebrae – to deliver pain-relieving medication directly to the site of inflammation.

Why they're used:

Epidural steroid injections have been used for almost half a century to treat **sciatica** (pain in the sciatic nerve, the major nerve of the leg, which runs from the lower end of the spine, behind the thigh and to the knee before dividing into smaller nerves). Your doctor may recommend an epidural steroid injection if you have acute sciatica or if ongoing pain makes it difficult to be active or do rehabilitation exercises.

How they're done:

Epidural steroids are administered at doctors' offices, clinics and at other outpatient facilities. If you and your doctor decide that an epidural steroid injection is appropriate, you can expect the procedure to last between 15 and 20 minutes.

Your doctor will have you lie flat on your stomach on an X-ray table. Before the actual injection into the epidural space, your doctor will inject a local anesthetic (pain-killing medication, similar to one used to numb your mouth prior to having a filling) into the area. Then, typically using an X-ray procedure called fluoroscopy, he or she will guide the needle into the epidural space and inject the steroid solution. After the injection, your doctor will probably want to monitor you for 15 to 20 minutes before allowing you to go home.

Once at home, you should take it easy for the rest of the day, but you may resume normal (that is, what's normal for you) activities the following day.

Prognosis:

By delivering medication directly to the site of inflammation, epidural steroid injections may ease pain in up to 50 percent of people who have the injections. Pain relief typically occurs in seven to 10 days and may last from a week to a year. Doctors may administer as many as three injections in six months' to a year's time.

SELECTIVE NERVE-ROOT BLOCK

When a nerve-root is compressed or inflamed, it can cause pain in the back and leg. A **selective nerve-root block** (SNRB) is an injection of a steroid and/or numbing agent into the area of the nerve where it exits the spinal column between the vertebrae.

Why they're used:

SNRBs are used in diagnosis. If an injection into a particular site relieves pain, the doctor can determine the source of the pain. SNRBs are also used for the treatment of back and leg pain, particularly pain from a herniated disc.

How they're done:

Like epidural steroid injections, selective nerve-root blocks are administered at doctors' offices, clinics and at other outpatient facilities. The procedure is performed under fluoroscopy, which enables the doctor to locate the precise space to be injected.

To have the procedure, you'll need to lie still on your stomach on an X-ray table while the doctor administers the injection. Although the injection itself will be mildly uncomfortable, if the site of pain has been correctly identified for injection, your nerve pain should start to improve quickly.

Your doctor will want to monitor you for a while before sending you home for a day's rest followed by normal, light activity.

Prognosis:

The success of the procedure lies largely on its ability to target the affected nerve root. If the nerve root injected is not the source of your pain, it will have no effect on your pain. In some cases, the injection itself may temporarily worsen pain.

If SNRB treatment is successful, your doctor may advise having up to three of these procedures per year, as needed.

FACET JOINT BLOCK

If your doctor suspects the source of your pain is in the facet joints, where the vertebrae connect to one another, he may recommend a procedure called a **facet joint block**, in which a steroid and/or anesthetic medication is injected directly into the joint capsule.

Why they're done:

Like SNRBs, facet joint blocks are used in diagnosis. If an injection into a particular site relieves pain, it can help the doctor determine the source of the pain. Facet joint blocks are also used as therapy for the treatment of pain resulting from injuries or from osteoarthritis affecting the facet joints, but there is little evidence of their effectiveness.

How they're done:

Like other spinal injections, facet joint blocks are performed on an out-patient basis under fluoroscopy.

To have the procedure, you'll need to lie flat on your stomach on an X-ray table while a specially trained doctor guides the needle into the facet joint suspected of causing your pain. Once the needle is in place, your doctor will inject the pain- and/or inflammation-easing medication into the facet joint capsule. If the facet joint was indeed the source of your pain, the anesthetic should provide some relief almost immediately, but you probably won't experience the full benefits of the procedure for about a week.

After the procedure, you will be monitored for a short while and then allowed to go home to rest for the remainder of the day. You should be able to resume light to normal activity the following day.

Prognosis:

As with selective nerve-root block, the effectiveness of facet joint blocks depends largely on whether the target of the injection was the actual cause of your back pain. If the injections are effective, your doctor may recommend having up to three procedures per year for sustained pain relief.

FACET NEUROTOMY

Facet neurotomy is a procedure that targets the nerve supplying the injured facet joint.

Why it's done:

For people in whom facet joint block has suggested that a particular joint is a cause of back pain, this procedure can provide longer relief than the injection of medication alone by disabling the nerve responsible for the pain.

How it's done:

Facet neurotomy is performed much like other spinal injections, in an outpatient setting. As you lie on your stomach on an X-ray table, your doctor will insert a needle into your affected facet joint, using fluoroscopy. Instead of injecting medication, however, the needle will contain a probe, which is then heated with radio waves and applied to the sensory nerve to the back, disrupting the nerve's ability to carry pain messages to the brain.

Prognosis:

Approximately half of those people with pain confirmed to result from problems with a facet joint find some lasting relief from facet neurotomy.

SACROILIAC JOINT BLOCK

Sacroiliac joint blocks are much like SNRBs and facet joint blocks, except that the anesthetic or anti-inflammatory medication is injected into the sacroiliac joint, which connects the sacrum (one of the lowest sections of the spine, composed of five fused vertebrae) to the pelvis.

Why it's done:

Like some other injections, sacroiliac joint blocks are used in diagnosis. When an injection brings pain relief, it helps confirm that the sacroiliac joint was a source of pain. Sacroiliac joint blocks are also used as therapy for low back pain that results from inflammation or damage within the sacroiliac joint.

How it's done:

Like many other injections used for back pain, sacroiliac joint block is performed on an outpatient basis under fluoroscopy. As you lie on your stomach on an X-ray table, a specially trained physician inserts a needle into the sacroiliac joint and injects a numbing agent and a steroid. After the procedure, you'll be monitored for a while before being allowed to go home.

Prognosis:

For the best results, sacroiliac joint block must be followed up by physical therapy and appropriate exercise to help keep the joint moving. If pain returns following sacroiliac joint block or if pain is not reduced to levels that make rehabilitation possible, the injections may be repeated up to three times per year.

PROLOTHERAPY

When surgery, medication and other conservative therapies have failed to bring back pain under control, some doctors recommend a procedure called **prolotherapy**. (Other names used for the prolotherapy procedure are sclerotherapy, regenerative injection therapy and nonsurgical ligament reconstruction.)

Unlike injections designed to ease inflammation, the goal of pro-lotherapy is to cause an inflammatory response through the injection of an irritant into injured soft tissues of the back. The reasoning is that the inflammation created will increase blood flow in tissues that are slow to heal because the blood flow to them is limited. In other words, the procedure sets in motion a healing process in small tears and weakened tissues that can lead to pain relief.

Although a handful of studies show some benefits of prolotherapy and some doctors swear by it, it is not widely practiced in the United States. It is not taught currently by conventional medical schools or hospital residency programs that physicians-in-training must complete.

Prolotherapy is most commonly performed by doctors, including anesthesiologists, orthopaedic surgeons, physiatrists and neurosurgeons, who have taken training courses offered by some professional organizations, such as the American Academy of Musculo-Skeletal Medicine and the American Association of Orthopaedic Medicine.

Why it's done:

Prolotherapy is used most commonly to ease back or neck pain associated with degenerative disc disease, sciatica or **whiplash** (damage to the ligaments, vertebrae, spinal cord or nerve-roots in the cervical spine caused by a sudden jerking back of the head and neck, such as in an auto accident).

How it's done:

The procedure is done on an outpatient basis, usually in a doctor's office. The doctor injects the irritant (a dextrose, or sugar, solution) into the affected tissues. Most people require four rounds to six rounds of injections to experience results, although some need fewer and some may require as many as 10.

Prognosis:

Many patients and physicians (including former U.S. Surgeon General C. Everett Koop) report pain relief using prolotherapy. But most of the support for its use is just that – reports, not scientific studies. Further research is needed to determine its use in the treatment of back pain and to compare its effectiveness with that of other therapies.

TRIGGER POINT INJECTIONS

The injection therapies we have discussed thus far involve injecting a medication or substance directly into the area of the spine. **Trigger point injections**, however, may be given throughout the muscular area of the back.

Trigger points are specific sites on the muscles that cause pain (both locally and throughout the back) when pressure is applied to them. You may have trigger points and not even be aware of them until your doctor presses on one during an exam. Trigger points are believed to occur due to excessive physical activity, fatigue or trauma.

Why they're done:

Trigger point injections, which involve injecting small amounts of a local anesthetic, sometimes along with a steroid medication, directly into painful trigger points, may be helpful for people who experience back pain when pressure is applied to certain areas.

How they're done:

Your doctor can give trigger point injections in his or her office or in an outpatient clinic. The procedure usually involves having between one injection and five injections using a fine needle. The entire procedure lasts between five and 15 minutes. Afterward, you'll be monitored for about an hour before you're allowed to go home and resume normal activity; however, you must be careful for the first few days to avoid excessive use of the injected muscles.

Prognosis:

Trigger point injections may be helpful in easing back pain for some people. Most doctors recommend using them on a short-term basis or during times when back pain is at its worst. If you decide to have trigger point injections, make sure that you do so along with other therapies – including oral medication therapies, exercise and physical therapy – that your doctor recommends.

THE BENEFITS AND RISKS OF INJECTIONS

Just like medications you take by mouth, injections can carry risks with their benefits. The risks vary by the specific procedure, but may be related to the substance injected or to the act of inserting the needle into the body.

Inserting needles required for these procedures has the potential to cause problems, such as infection, bleeding or even nerve damage, although such problems are rare. A risk of epidural injections, in particular, is a puncture of the dura, which may cause some spinal fluid to leak. Although the puncture itself isn't serious, it can cause a headache that may last up to a few days. Like other side effects of injections, a dural puncture is rare.

Still, it's important to speak to your physician about the risks and benefits of any procedure you are considering and to weigh them carefully with your physician before making a treatment decision.

Implantable Pain Relief Devices

There are two basic types of implantable devices for pain relief: those that deliver electrical stimulation to the spinal cord and those that deliver medication to it.

SPINAL CORD STIMULATION

Since the 1960s, electricity has been used in the treatment of leg pain. Spinal cord stimulation (SCS) is believed to decrease the perception of pain by activating nerves in your lower back to block pain signals going to that area. As a result, pain is replaced with a pleasant tingling sensation.

SCS is delivered through a set of electrodes that are inserted between the vertebrae into the epidural space. A pulse generator or radio receiver surgically placed under the skin in the abdomen or the upper buttock area activates the electrodes.

Why it's done:

SCS may be appropriate for people with nerve-root injuries that haven't responded to conventional treatments or for people for whom surgery – sometimes multiple surgeries – to correct the cause of leg pain has not been successful. SCS is not useful for back pain itself.

How it's done:

Implantation of an SCS device is done in at least two stages, usually in a hospital. The first step involves placing a "trial" lead or wire containing a set of electrodes into the epidural space through a catheter inserted through a small puncture in the back. For this stage of the procedure, you'll probably have a course of intravenous sedation and local anesthesia. The lead is then connected to a small electrical device, called a stimulator, which is about the size of a silver dollar.

At least initially, you'll be sent home with a temporary, external device. If, after a few days, you decide the device doesn't help much, the device and wires that lead to your spine can be removed without additional surgery. If you find the device helpful, on the other hand, you can opt to have it placed in your body during a second procedure.

The second stage takes about 90 minutes and is performed under local anesthetic. Your doctor will need you to be awake to help him or her appropriately place the electrodes to provide maximum relief. After the procedure, you will be observed for a while and given instructions on how to operate the device. Most people are allowed to go home the same day of surgery.

Prognosis:

Long term, as many as 60 percent of people with SCS are satisfied with the level of pain relief they get from SCS; however, few experience complete pain relief.

IMPLANTED DRUG INFUSION

Implanted drug infusion (intraspinal drug infusion therapy) is much like SCS, except that it uses medication, not electrical stimulation, to ease pain.

Intraspinal drug infusion therapy involves implanting a "pump" in the body to deliver a regular, predetermined dose of pain medication via a thin tube into the painful area of the spine. By targeting medication to the precise site of pain, the device enables you to use much smaller amounts of medication than would otherwise be necessary to control pain. Precise targeting of small doses also reduces the risk of side effects you might experience from higher oral doses of pain-relieving medication.

Why it's done:

Intraspinal drug infusion therapy usually is reserved for people who have pain primarily in their lower back and buttocks that hasn't responded to more conservative treatment options. Like spinal cord stimulation, it may be appropriate for people for whom surgery – sometimes multiple surgeries – to correct the cause of back pain has not been successful.

How it's done:

The procedure to implant a medication pump is much like that used for SCS. As with SCS, a trial pump that stays outside the body is used first to deliver pain medication through a tube inserted into the affected area of the spine. If you find that the pump is helpful, your doctor can permanently implant it.

Prognosis:

If other pain relief treatments have failed and you meet the criteria for intraspinal drug infusion therapy, this therapy may help you bring pain to a more tolerable level. Be aware that the procedure involves more than just implanting a device. It requires a commitment to continue other pain-relief therapies, such as exercise and physical therapy as well as lifestyle modifications.

It also requires a commitment for regular doctor visits to keep the pump delivering its medication. At least once every few months, you'll have to have your pump refilled with medication. The simple procedure involves injecting medication through your skin into the pump's reservoir.

The Benefits and Risks of Implanted Devices

Like all medical treatments, implanted devices carry some risks. Fortunately, in most cases, these risks are minor, and include possible infection of the injection site and, in the case of drug infusion, drug side effects.

A TREATMENT OF (ALMOST) LAST RESORT

Because placing implantable devices requires surgery and doesn't actually correct the problem causing the pain, doctors don't recommend them for anyone who hasn't exhausted more conservative treatments, including, in many cases, conventional surgery to correct the problem. (See Chapter 5, "Pain Relief Through Surgery.") Other factors that will influence your doctor's decision to prescribe implantable devices include the following:

Your symptoms. If the symptoms you're experiencing aren't consistent with the results of diagnostic tests, there may be factors at play in your pain that an implanted device won't relieve. In those cases, continuing to look for the source of the pain, rather than mask the pain with an electronic device, might be a wiser choice.

The role of emotions in your pain. If your doctor suspects that your pain may be largely influenced by depression or anxiety, an implanted device probably won't help much. In fact, your insurance company may require that you have a psychological evaluation before agreeing to cover the implantation of a device. In this case, you might need to explore stress-relief techniques or even medications that may help you control your anxiety or depression.

Your willingness to continue other therapies. Implanted devices work best in conjunction with conservative therapies. Back pain always requires treatment integrating exercise, healthy lifestyle habits, rest, stress reduction and other strategies, which we'll discuss later in the book. If you aren't willing to try or to continue these other components of therapy, you probably aren't the best candidate for an implanted device.

Nevertheless, if you meet the criteria outlined in the descriptions of the specific therapies, and if you are committed to continuing exercise, physical therapy and other pain-relief therapies while using the implanted devices, implantable devices may be just what you need to get your pain under control.

What if your back pain is the result of a problem that can be corrected surgically? In that case, correcting the actual problem – rather than just easing your symptoms as implantable therapies do – usually makes more sense. In the next chapter, we'll discuss common back surgeries and when these operations can be helpful.

chapter 5:

Pain Relief Through Surgery

What if medications don't ease your back pain? What if your back pain persists and gets worse? Your next option may be back surgery. In other cases, surgery may be your best – or only – option from the start.

Making the decision to have back surgery, and having a successful surgery and recovery, is not easy. You won't – and can't – do this alone. You and your doctor will have to determine if back surgery is the right course for your condition. You, your employer and your family or other support system will have to work together to make sure that your surgery, recovery and rehabilitation go smoothly. Back surgery is a serious endeavor that requires a commitment from you and others in your life.

In this chapter, we'll take a look at some of the different medical problems that may warrant surgery and some of the various types of surgery to relieve those problems. We'll also look at some of the issues you should consider and questions you should ask your doctor – and yourself – before you commit to any type of surgery.

When Is Back Surgery Necessary?

If you have a problem that can be corrected, such as a herniated disc, spinal stenosis or spondylolisthesis, surgery is certainly an option worth considering – particularly when more conservative treatments, such as medical therapies and exercise, fail to relieve your pain. To treat certain other problems – such as a serious infection, tumor or a cauda equina syndrome – back surgery may be a medical necessity.

For the vast majority of problems that cause back pain, however, surgery isn't necessary or even useful. Most cases of back pain respond to medications, conservative non-medication therapies (see Chapter 6, "Beyond Medicine and Surgery," and Chapter 7, "Another Way," for some of these other therapies) and the simple passage of time.

For this reason, many physicians agree that surgery should be a treatment of last resort. Most doctors will recommend surgery only after other options have failed to help.

Still, for people with some back problems, surgery can bring effective or long-lasting relief. Surgical procedures available today, for example, can ease herniated discs, remove material that narrows the spine and presses on nerves, and bolster fractured vertebrae.

Most Common Surgeries

Back surgery is most commonly performed for one of three medical problems: herniated discs, spinal stenosis and spondylolisthesis. In the following section, we'll discuss the most common surgeries to treat these problems.

DISCECTOMY

Discectomy is the removal of part of a disc that is herniated and causing pain. Most discectomies performed in this country are referred to as either arthroscopic or microsurgical. Let's explore these two types now.

Percutaneous Discectomy

Percutaneous (meaning through the skin) discectomy involves removing a portion of a herniated disc, using a laser or suction device, through a narrow probe placed into your back. In many cases, removing the injured disc relieves the pressure the disc places on the nerves, thereby easing pain.

Why it's done:

Although not all discs that are herniated need to be removed, for some people, removal of the disc is beneficial when other therapies don't help. Discectomy may be advised if a herniated disc causes sciatica (pain running down the leg) or scoliosis, a condition in which muscle spasms cause a curvature of the spine. Discectomy may be medically necessary if a herniated disc compresses nerves critical to bowel and bladder function, resulting in the rare condition cauda equina syndrome.

How it's done:

Percutaneous discectomy is performed under local anesthesia (to learn more about the different types of anesthesia, see "Anesthesia: To Sleep or Not To Sleep" on page 92) in an outpatient procedure.

To perform a percutaneous discectomy, the surgeon places a probe, guided by fluoroscopy (a procedure in which X-ray images of the body are displayed on a fluorescent screen), into the affected disc. Tiny surgical instruments are then placed down the hollow center of the probe to remove injured portions of the disc. Once the damage is removed, the surgeon removes the probe and places a bandage over the puncture site, which is no larger in diameter than a pencil eraser. No stitches are needed.

The procedure typically takes about an hour and is, at most, mildly painful. After being observed in the recovery room for a few hours, you will be allowed to go home and resume limited activities the next day.

Prognosis:

For many people who have pain or numbness caused by herniated discs, discectomy is a useful treatment. If you undergo discectomy, be prepared to experience some minor, temporary discomforts – including a tingling sensation and possible muscle spasms in the treated part of the spine – after surgery. It's also important that you faithfully perform any back exercises your doctor or physical therapist recommends during your recovery. Consult your doctor before resuming sports or vigorous activity. Typically, it will be three to four weeks before you can resume your previous level of activity.

Microsurgical Discectomy

Microsurgical discectomy requires a small incision, usually less than an inch long. During this type of discectomy, the surgeon, using a microscope, removes the damaged portion of the disc along with a small portion of the bone covering the spinal canal.

Why it's done:

Microsurgical discectomy may be advised if a herniated disc causes sciatica or weakness that interferes with your daily function, or if you have more than one herniated disc. Because only a small incision is used, it is still a minimally painful procedure. It may correct more extensive damage than can be achieved by percutaneous discectomy.

How it's done:

Microsurgical discectomy is performed under general anesthesia in a hospital operating room. To perform a microsurgical discectomy, the surgeon makes a small incision in your back. Then, using a piece of equipment that magnifies the small structures of the spine, he or she removes the damaged disc or discs, sometimes along with small portions of bone covering the spinal column that are contributing to pain and/or weakness. Depending on the extent of the damage being corrected, the procedure may last from 45 minutes to several hours.

While the pain of microdiscectomy typically is more than that of percutaneous discectomy, it is generally mild and highly controllable with pain medications. You should be able to go home the day after surgery and resume sedentary or light activity.

Prognosis:

For people who have pain or problems related to herniated discs, microsurgical discectomy is often an effective treatment option. But like any surgery, it is not a cure-all, and it doesn't work for everyone. The localized pain following surgery usually resolves in a matter of days, but sciatica, if that was the reason for the surgery, may linger for a month or more before improving. Because the damaged disc is not completely removed during the procedure, it is possible (though not common) for the disc to grow back, often necessitating a second surgery.

LAMINECTOMY

When spinal stenosis, a narrowing of the spinal column, causes pressure on the nerve roots, one option is enlarging the spinal column to make more room for the affected nerves through a procedure called **laminectomy**.

Laminectomy specifically involves removing the lamina, the back-side of the spinal canal that forms a roof over the spinal cord. Along with the lamina, doctors often remove any bony protrusions, called spurs, which may have formed as a result of osteoarthritis of the spine.

Why it's done:

Laminectomy usually is done when more conservative treatments fail to relieve painful nerve compression associated with spinal stenosis.

How it's done:

Laminectomy is a major surgical procedure performed in a hospital under general anesthesia. To perform a laminectomy, the surgeon makes an incision down the center of the affected section of the back – usually the lumbar, or lower, section – and then moves the muscles to one side.

Once the spine is visible, your surgeon will examine the vertebrae. He or she may also take an X-ray to determine which vertebrae are problematic. Once the surgeon has determined the problem, he or she can remove lamina and bone spurs.

Prognosis:

In selected cases, laminectomy can be useful in relieving pain and restoring strength and sensation to areas affected by compressed nerves. But the procedure is not without risks (See "Is Surgery an Option for Me?" on page 85), and recovery can take some time.

After the procedure, you'll probably need to stay in the hospital for at least a couple of days and you may want to consider spending an additional week, or even several weeks, in a rehabilitation facility. For best results, you'll need to undergo physical therapy, beginning a week or two after surgery. Complete recovery may take several months.

SPINAL FUSION

Spinal fusion is a welding process by which two or more vertebrae are fused together to form a single immobile unit.

Why it's done:

Spinal fusion is used to stop the motion that normally occurs between vertebrae. It may be used to relieve pain that is caused or aggravated by movements such as bending, lifting or twisting, or to stabilize a spine that has been damaged by infections or tumors. It may also be used to stop the progression of a spinal deformity, such as scoliosis, to treat injuries to the vertebrae or to stabilize vertebrae that become loose due to a defect in the facet joint.

How it's done:

Spinal fusion is major surgery performed in a hospital under general anesthesia. The procedure often requires two surgeries – one to remove bone from another site of the body, such as the hip or pelvis, the other on the spine itself.

Your surgeon will use small pieces of your own bone or, sometimes, bone donated from another person, to fill the spaces between the affected vertebrae and promote the vertebrae's growth. After putting such bone grafts into place, your surgeon will then immobilize the adjacent segments of the spine to allow the fusion to progress. He or she may use devices such as metal rods or screws to keep your spine from moving while the vertebrae grow together.

Prognosis:

If you have problems related to unstable vertebrae, spinal fusion can be an effective procedure, but it should be considered carefully. While most fusions are successful, the recovery time can be long and the rehabilitation process difficult.

If you are a smoker, it's important to stop smoking prior to undergoing fusion. Studies have shown that smokers are significantly less likely to have a successful fusion than nonsmokers.

NEWER OPTIONS:
VERTEBROPLASTY AND KYPHOPLASTY

While herniated discs, spinal stenosis and unstable vertebrae are the most common reasons for back surgery, they are not the only reasons. In recent years, doctors have begun using two new and similar surgical procedures, **vertebroplasty** and **kyphoplasty**, to relieve the pain and, possibly, other problems associated with compression fractures of the vertebrae.

A compression fracture occurs when a vertebra becomes so thin and damaged from osteoporosis that it can no longer support the weight above it. As a result, it crumbles and compresses, often to about half its height, and may cause the spine to shift forward at the fracture site.

Why they're done:

Both vertebroplasty and kyphoplasty are typically performed by orthopaedic surgeons or specialists called interventional radiologists. These procedures involve bolstering fractured bone with a cement-like material that is administered through a minimally invasive surgical procedure.

How they're done:

To administer the material, a physician first makes a small incision in the skin over the fractured vertebra or vertebrae. He or she then inserts a needle about as big around as a cocktail straw. Using special imaging equipment, the doctor is able to direct the needle right into the fractured vertebrae.

Although the two procedures are essentially the same, kyphoplasty involves an additional step. Just before injecting the cement-like material, the doctor places a small, balloon-like device into the compressed vertebra and inflates it. The goal of the additional step is to help restore height to the crumbled vertebra, which will reduce deformity.

For most people, the procedure requires only a mild sedative. It is performed on an outpatient basis, and most people are able to return home within a few hours after the procedure.

Prognosis:

Both vertebroplasty and kyphoplasty may be effective in relieving pain of vertebral fractures that doesn't go away on its own. Kyphoplasty may have the additional benefit of helping to prevent kyphosis, the forward curvature of the spine that is common in people – especially women – who've had osteoporotic fractures of the vertebrae. Because both procedures are relatively new and still under review by the FDA, little is known about their long-term effectiveness and safety.

Is Surgery an Option for Me?

Once you've exhausted more conservative treatments, such as medications, physical therapy and possibly injection therapies, your doctor and a surgeon will help you determine if surgery – and if so, what type of surgery – might help you.

You will play a major role in that decision, because in most cases of back pain, the decision to have surgery is a personal judgment call. Are you willing to undergo major surgery and weeks or months of rehabilitation for the prospect of having less pain and improved function? Would you undergo the risks of surgery for the opportunity to live day-to-day with little or no pain medication?

As you consider whether or not to have surgery, keep in mind that every person's situation is different. You may not benefit from the same surgery that a friend, family member or the majority of participants in a medical study did. Your doctor may advise against a particular surgery or warn you that its chances of success are low. Even if your doctor thinks that surgery can help you, there are still many factors that both you and your doctor must consider, including the following:

Other health problems. If you have heart disease or lung disease, the strain of some types of surgery may be too much for you. Before having any kind of surgery, it's important to have other health problems under control.

Unhealthy habits. If you smoke or consume large amounts of alcohol, you need to address these problems before surgery. Both smoking and excessive alcohol intake can interfere with bone growth and healing. Any unhealthy habits can interfere with the success of surgery and lengthen the time it takes to recover from it.

Your medications. In some cases, you may need to stop some of the medications you are taking for a while prior to surgery. For example, aspirin and other nonsteroidal anti-inflammatory drugs, which you may be taking to ease pain and inflammation, may interfere with blood clotting and cause you to bleed excessively during surgery.

On the other hand, glucocorticoid medications such as prednisone may be needed at larger doses during surgery. The reason is that these drugs are similar to hormones our bodies naturally produce in response to stress. In people who take synthetic glucocorticoids, the body's ability to increase its own production of these hormones may be hampered. Therefore, additional medication may be necessary to help your body meet the demands of the situation.

Infections. If you have any type of bacterial infection in your body (even an abscessed tooth), you'll need to have it cleared up before you undergo any surgery. One possible problem after joint surgery is infection, which can spread from another part of your body to your joint through the bloodstream.

Your weight. If you are overweight, it's best to start losing pounds before you decide to have surgery. Being overweight may put extra stress on your heart and lungs during surgery. Excess weight can be hard on your back as well and it can make it more difficult for you to do the exercises you'll need to do as you recover.

Even a modest loss of 10 percent of your body weight can make a difference, but for many people even losing a small amount of weight takes a well-designed diet and exercise program as well as commitment and willpower. Consult your physician if you're not sure if you need to lose weight or, if you do need to lose, how to best go about it. The Arthritis Foundation publishes a new book with weight-loss guidance and motivation, *Change Your Life! Simple Strategies to Lose Weight, Get Fit and*

Improve Your Outlook. Call 800/207-8633 or log on to www.arthritis.org to find out more about this book and other Arthritis Foundation resources.

Strength and fitness. Although any rehabilitation program after surgery will involve performing exercises to strengthen the muscles of the back, doing such exercises beforehand may increase your odds of surgical success. Similarly, aerobic exercise can prepare your heart and lungs for the rigors of surgery and rehabilitation. To learn more about what you can do to improve your physical fitness prior to surgery, consult your doctor or physical therapist.

Your care as you recuperate. One of your major concerns as you consider surgery may not be getting through the surgery, but caring for yourself in the days and weeks that follow. Things to consider if you are having a major procedure, such as a laminectomy or spinal fusion, include: Who will care for your home, children, pets, plants, etc., while you are in the hospital? Who will care for you once you are home?

Depending on the type of surgery you have, it may be a few days or a couple of months before you are able to do things like stand for prolonged periods, drive a car, vacuum or shower without the assistance of another adult. Consider your personal support systems – or the possibility or hiring someone to help you for a while – before you schedule surgery.

If you properly prepare for surgery, you'll have less to do or be concerned about when the time arrives, and relieving yourself of that stress now may actually help you recuperate faster. Nevertheless, recovering from surgery – particularly major surgery – requires you to make a major commitment. The amount of work you put into a recovery process often makes the difference between success and failure and decreases your risk of adverse effects. In general, here's what you can expect to do following major joint surgery.

Work your muscles. Following surgery, and maybe even before the procedure, your doctor will likely refer you to a physical therapist. This health-care professional will give you a program of exercises that will help strengthen the muscles that support your spine. It's important that you fol-

When Surgery Is a Necessity

Though you may think otherwise when you're in pain, back surgery is rarely a life-and-death matter. In most cases, you'll have months – or even years – to weigh the risks and benefits of surgery, try other treatments, consider alternatives and consult a surgeon.

If you have one of the following, however, back surgery may be essential:

CAUDA EQUINA SYNDROME. In this rare condition, nerve roots that supply the bladder and bowel along with the groin and anal areas, are compressed, leading to loss of sensation, sexual function and ability to urinate. Without surgery to relieve compression on these nerve roots, cauda equina syndrome could become permanent.

A TUMOR. Even a noncancerous (or benign) tumor can press on important areas of the spine, necessitating the tumor's removal. Some tumors can be left alone, however. An experienced surgeon can advise you.

AN INFECTION. Infections can enter virtually any part of your body, including (in rare cases) your spine. If antibiotics fail to clear a spinal infection, surgery may be necessary to clear away infected areas.

low the program faithfully, even when it may be painful to do so, to gain as much use of the joint as possible. Exercise will begin gradually and become progressively more strenuous as your joint gains strength and mobility.

Heed limits. As you start to feel better, you may be tempted to do too much too soon. Resist this temptation. Putting excess stress on your vulnerable back can cause damage and possibly necessitate further surgery. While exercise is essential, attempting to lift heavy loads or engage in vigorous activities soon after any spinal surgery is unwise. To find out how much you can do and how soon, consult your doctor.

Take your medications. It's important that you take any medications your doctor prescribes exactly as directed. Medications you may need following surgery include narcotic analgesics to relieve pain and make it easier to perform your exercises; blood thinners to reduce the risk of blood clots; antibiotics to reduce infection risk and, of course, any medications you need to keep other medical problems you might have under control.

Steer clear of infection. Even after you've recovered from surgery, it's important that you take extra precautions against bacterial infection, particularly if you have devices such as rods or screws implanted in your spine. For example, if you cut your finger on a kitchen knife or step on a nail, it's important that you ask your doctor about a course of antibiotics. Any infection that enters the body through the bloodstream may settle in the joint, causing problems that may require further surgery to correct.

By properly preparing for back surgery, following doctors' orders and using common sense afterwards, your surgery may offer a lifetime of pain relief and increased mobility. However, as with any surgery, back surgery offers no guarantees. In rare instances, surgery can lead to infection, damaged discs can grow back to cause more pain, blood vessels or nerves can be damaged, fused bone can refuse to weld together and scarring after surgery can cause pain. All of these factors and possible situations must be considered as you make the decision whether or not to have surgery.

Preparing for Surgery

Because of the potential risks, no surgery performed for any reason should be taken lightly. You'll want to know as much as you can about the surgery – and any possible alternatives – before committing to it.

Most surgeries for back pain are considered elective (in other words, they aren't performed under emergency or life-and-death circumstances), so you'll have some time to carefully weigh your decision. (To learn about cases when surgery is a must, see "When Surgery Is a Necessity" on page 88.)

Unless your surgery is urgent, you'll have time to seek out a surgeon with whom you feel comfortable (for advice on finding a surgeon, see "Finding the Right Surgeon" page 94) and question him or her about your need for surgery and results you can expect. **Following are questions you'll want to ask as you contemplate surgery.**

- What other kinds of treatment could I have instead of surgery?
- How successful might those treatments be?
- Can you explain this surgical procedure, step by step?
- May I view materials or videos of this surgery?
- How long does this surgery typically take?
- Do you offer a class or informational meeting for people considering this surgery? (Some hospitals do.)
- May I have this surgery on an outpatient basis?
- What are the risks involved in the surgery? How likely are they?
- How can I avoid blood transfusions? What other options are there?
- What type of anesthesia will be used? What are the risks of anesthesia?
- How much improvement can I expect from the surgery?

- Will more surgery be necessary? After what period of time?
- If I choose to undergo this surgery, will you contact my family doctor?
- Will he or she be involved in my hospital stay?
- If so, in what way?
- Are you board-certified?
- What is your experience doing this type of surgery?
- What is the hospital's experience with this type of surgery?
- Can you give me the name of someone else who has undergone this surgery and who would talk to me about it?
- Is an exercise program recommended before and after the operation?
- Must I stop taking – or increase the dosage of – any of my medications before surgery?
- What happens if I delay surgery? Even for a few months?
- What are the risks if I don't have the surgery?

If you decide to proceed with surgery, here are some more questions you will want to ask your doctor. You may also wish to look over your insurance policy, if you have one, to be aware of your coverage for surgery.

- How long will I need to stay in the hospital after having the surgery?
- How much pain is involved? Will I receive medication for it? What kind of pain is normal to expect? How long will this pain last?
- How long do I have to stay in bed?
- When will I start physical therapy? Will I need home or outpatient therapy?
- Will in-hospital rehabilitation be covered by my insurance?
- May I review written material or videotapes about this phase of my care?
- Are physical therapy, occupational therapy and home health care covered by my insurance? For how long? (You may need to ask your insur-

ance company about this issue and have someone confirm up front what it will pay. Also, be aware that some insurance companies require a second opinion before authorizing any elective surgery.)

- Will I need to arrange for some assistance at home? If so, for how long?
- Will I need any special equipment for my home? Will I need to make any modifications to my home?
- What medications will I need for my recovery? How long will I need to take them?
- What limits will there be on my activities – driving, using the toilet, climbing stairs, bending, eating, having sex?
- How often will I have follow-up visits with you? Are they included in the cost of the surgery?

You may also find it helpful to talk to another person with your type of back problem who has already had the surgery you are considering. Your doctor may be able to refer you to another patient. Some of the questions outlined here might be appropriate to ask that person, too. Remember: Every person and every surgery is different. Your surgery may not go exactly as another person's, even though your situations are similar.

Anesthesia: To Sleep or Not To Sleep

Regardless of the type of surgery you have, it's almost a certainty that you will need some type of anesthesia. While most people associate anesthesia purely with pain relief, it has an additional purpose in the operating room. Anesthesia allows your surgeon and his or her team to control a wide range of natural bodily reflexes, such as heart rate and blood pressure, which could fluctuate dangerously in response to the trauma of surgery.

Your doctor will recommend one of three types of anesthesia – general, regional or local – to block your pain and control your natural bodily reflexes. Here's a brief overview of these three types of anesthesia.

GENERAL ANESTHESIA

Having general anesthesia is often referred to as being "put to sleep." General anesthesia temporarily stops the brain's overall ability to sense and remember pain. Under general anesthesia, which you breathe in through a face mask, you are asleep. When you awaken, you may have vivid memories of the hours and minutes leading up to surgery. You may even remember being wheeled into the operating room and being asked to count backwards as the anesthetic puts you to sleep. But you will have no recollection of the time you are asleep or of the surgery itself.

LOCAL OR REGIONAL ANESTHESIA

With both local and regional anesthesia, on the other hand, you are fully aware of what is going on during surgery and will remember the surgery.

With local anesthesia, the doctor blocks the pain signal where the nerve begins; only a small, specific area of the body is numbed. Often, a doctor will use an intravenous sedative along with local anesthetic to help ease anxiety and enable you to relax and stay still during the surgery.

Regional anesthesia involves blocking pain responses from an entire region of the body, by injecting an anesthetic into the outer covering of the spinal column (called epidural anesthesia). If you were undergoing lower back surgery, for example, your doctor might block pain signals from your waist down. You would still have full feeling in your upper body and even be able to speak with the surgical staff during the actual procedure.

WHICH ANESTHESIA IS BEST?

When it comes to back surgery, the specific type of surgery you have will largely dictate the type of anesthesia you receive. Longer, more involved surgeries usually require general anesthesia. For shorter, less complicated surgeries, general anesthesia typically isn't necessary. In fact, your doctor may want you to stay awake so that you play a role in the surgery.

Other benefits of local or regional anesthesia are that they are gen-

Finding the Right Surgeon

If you have a back problem that may require surgery, it's important that you find the best doctor to do the job. In most cases, you'll want to consult more than one surgeon before committing to surgery. To locate good prospects, try the following strategies:

Ask your primary-care physician for a referral. He or she is in a good position to know which doctors are available in your area.

Ask friends and family members. Chances are good that someone you know has had back problems. If they've had a good experience with a doctor, they will probably be more than happy to pass along this name. But keep in mind that all people and all surgeries are different. The best doctor for that person may not be the best for you.

Consult your insurer. Ask your insurance carrier to provide a list of doctors who perform the type of surgery you need. In some cases, your insurance may limit your choice of doctors.

Check with a referral service. Many universities will refer you to doctors who are associated with their hospitals and medical centers.

Check with professional organizations. Many professional org-

erally less risky and you recover from them more quickly. Also, by avoiding the grogginess that comes with general anesthesia, you may be able to be up and active sooner, which may improve the odds of long-term success of the procedure.

Nevertheless, there are situations where general anesthesia is necessary. By considering the type of surgery, your health and your preferences, your doctor may recommend the appropriate anesthesia choice for you.

anizations for physicians can give you the names of doctors in your area. For more information on these resources, see "Which Doctor Should You See?" on page 20.

Once you have the names of several doctors, find out as much as you can about each one. Do they specialize in spinal surgery? How many spinal surgeries have they performed? What kind of training have they had in spinal surgery? The doctor's professional organization or practice may be able to provide the information you need.

Once you have identified your top choices, pick one or two doctors to meet personally. The doctor you choose should be one who:

- Welcomes your questions and tries his or her best to answer them;
- Is willing to discuss both the risks and benefits of the surgery he or she is recommending;
- Encourages you to get a second opinion if you feel you need it;
- Is willing to discuss conservative alternatives to surgery; and
- Makes you feel comfortable and confident in his or her abilities.

chapter 6

Beyond Medication and Surgery: Non-Medical Treatments

As we have discussed, the vast majority of back problems never require surgery. Many don't require strong medication or taking medication long-term. While medications may be of help in easing short-term pain, and surgery may be useful in correcting certain painful problems, the answer to controlling ongoing pain, in most cases, lies in a variety of non-medical, non-surgical therapies. A physician or other health-care professional usually administers some of these therapies, but others you can do on your own.

If your health-care provider doesn't recommend non-drug therapies, bring up the subject yourself. Ask questions about which ones might be appropriate for you, and then follow up! Be an effective self-manager. We'll discuss how you can do this in the next section.

What Is an Effective Self-Manager?

People who manage best with chronic pain are what health professionals call effective self-managers. That is, instead of passively following their doctors' orders – and nothing more – these people take an active role in their own health care.

Effective self-managers have a give-and-take with their doctor and other providers. They work at keeping healthy lifestyles, read up on health advances and ask their doctors about new therapies. They take their medications as prescribed and undergo surgery if necessary, but they don't stop there. They are open to the non-surgical, non-drug therapies, many of which they can try on their own.

The following therapies are some you may find helpful as you work with your doctor to manage your pain. Even if your situation requires medication or surgery, the addition of non-surgical, non-drug therapies is essential to get the most out of your treatment.

In this chapter, we'll discuss some of the most commonly prescribed or used pain therapies. Your own doctor may recommend a combination of these. Many of them you can do on your own; however, it's always best to consult a health professional before starting any kind of treatment.

PHYSICAL THERAPY

Taught and/or administered by a health-care professional called a **physical therapist** (PT), physical therapy is a rehabilitation program focusing largely on exercises to strengthen the muscles in your back. Your doctor may recommend physical therapy to strengthen a bad back, which can help prevent recurrences of pain or help you recover from back surgery.

The college course work required to complete a physical therapy degree includes basic science courses, such as biology, chemistry and physics, and more specialized courses, such as manifestations of disease, examination techniques and therapeutic procedures. To practice, degreed physical therapists must pass a licensure exam in their state.

The exercises you will perform in physical therapy as well as their frequency and duration will depend largely on your goals. If the goal is to recover some of your spine's flexibility after surgery or immobilization, a few weeks to a few months of physical therapy may be sufficient. If your goal is to keep abdominal muscles strong to prevent recurrences of back pain, you may want to keep up your PT-prescribed exercises indefinitely.

In addition to the strengthening exercises, a physical therapist may use or recommend other therapies, including massage (some PTs are licensed to perform massage), ultrasound, and hot and cold packs, which we'll discuss in more detail later in this chapter.

WATER THERAPY

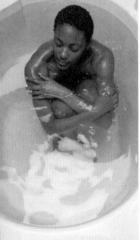

You know how good it can feel to soak in a warm tub, especially when your back is aching. It turns out that being in water not only feels good, it's good for you. Studies have shown that the benefits of applying heat (see "Hot and Cold Treatments" on page 102) can include muscle relaxation and decreased pain and stiffness. Immersing your body in warm water is an especially good way to apply heat to many parts of the body – all at once.

By allowing your muscles to relax, warm water also provides an excellent environment for exercise. Furthermore, water may act as resistance to help build muscle strength during exercise, and if back problems make it difficult to exercise, the buoyancy of water makes it easier and allows you to move in ways that you can't achieve outside of the water.

If you find that pain and stiffness are worst in the morning, soaking and/or performing gentle exercises in a tub, whirlpool bath or warm shower upon rising can help get you ready to take on your daily activities. (For some examples of warm-water exercises you can do right in your tub or whirlpool bath, see page 113.) If pain increases through the day, a warm soak before bedtime might make it easier to get to sleep.

Be aware that some people find soaking before bedtime to be stimulating, and this practice keeps them awake. If that's the case with you, limit your use of warm water to the afternoon and early evening hours.

Hot Tub Safety Tips

Warm water can work wonders on sore backs, but like any therapy, it should be used with care. When soaking in a hot tub or whirlpool, follow these safety tips:

- If you have difficulty getting in and out of the tub, try to use it only when someone else is around to help you.
- Check with your doctor before using a hot tub if you have any special medical conditions, such as lung or heart disease, circulatory problems, high or low blood pressure, diabetes, multiple sclerosis, skin irritations or any other serious illness.
- Check the thermometer for appropriate temperature before entering and while in the tub. Most experts recommend keeping the temperature around 104 degrees. Higher temperatures can increase your risk of fainting.
- If you start feeling light-headed or nauseated, get out of the water immediately.
- If swelling, stiffness or pain increase, discontinue use and consult your doctor.
- Don't use a hot tub during or after drinking alcohol or using narcotic analgesics.
- Don't use a hot tub if you are pregnant without first consulting your doctor.

MASSAGE THERAPY

Who couldn't benefit from a good back rub? It's no surprise that massage therapy is one of the most widely used therapies for back pain. Many doctors recommend it for their patients, and some doctors even have massage therapists working in their clinics.

Although there are many forms of massage, the type most people are familiar with is Swedish massage, a full body treatment that involves stroking or kneading the top layers of muscles with oils or lotions. Other forms of massage include:

- **Deep-tissue massage**, in which the massage therapist uses fingers, thumbs and even elbows to put strong pressure on deep muscle or tissue layers to relieve chronic tension.
- **Neuromuscular massage (also called trigger point therapy)**, in which the therapist uses his or her fingers to apply pressure to certain spots that can trigger pain in other parts of the body.
- **Myofascial release**, a type of massage that involves applying slow, steady pressure to relieve tension in the fascia, or thin tissue around the muscles.

Although massage therapy is generally safe, as with any therapy, you should take some precautions. For example, you should never have massage on an inflamed joint or on skin that is broken or infected. Let your massage therapist know if you have other health problems, including circulatory problems such as high blood pressure.

If you think you might be interested in massage, consult your physician, physical therapist or other health professional who may be able to refer you to a massage therapist with experience in your particular condition.

If you have a condition other than a common sprain or strain that causes pain, it's important that you see a massage therapist who is familiar with and has experience massaging people with your condition. A disease such as ankylosing spondylitis or osteoporosis of the spine may require special precautions.

How To Do Self-Massage

Ouch! You bump your (not so) funny bone or pinch your finger in the front door. What is your first response? If you're like most people, you probably rub the painful area. When you do, it probably feels a little better, at least for a while.

With a little instruction and practice, a similar type of rubbing – called self-massage – can help relieve back pain. Because your back is, well, behind you, you may not be able to do all of your massaging with your hands. If you'd like to try self-massage, here are a few suggestions (including some methods that use household items) to use in place of fingers:

Get professional advice. A massage therapist can show you some techniques to use yourself.

Warm up before you start. A warm bath or shower can relax you, make your hands more limber and improve circulation.

Create a healing environment. Find a warm, quiet place without distractions. For some people, music can help create a relaxing environment.

Use a little lotion. Using a little oil or lotion can help your hands glide over your body. A lightly scented massage oil can be soothing to your body – and your spirit.

Protect your spine. If you have back problems, placing pressure directly on your back could be harmful.

Have a ball. If you have trouble reaching beyond the tops of

continued on page 102

continued from page 101

your shoulders or sides of your lower back, see if you can find a friend or partner to help. If that's not possible, try using a tennis ball or other soft rubber ball. Lie on your back on the floor, place the ball under the painful area of your back and roll around.

Roll with it. If rolling on the floor sounds difficult or unappealing, try soothing your aching back with a massaging device purchased from a medical supply store or even a common paint roller. Many specialty stores offer massaging devices. A physical therapist should be able to recommend a good device and show you how to use it.

HOT AND COLD TREATMENTS

Using heat and cold treatments, easy relief methods you can do at home, can temporarily reduce back pain and stiffness. Cold packs can numb the painful area and reduce inflammation and swelling. They are especially good for back pain caused by injuries. Heat, on the other hand, relaxes muscles and stimulates blood circulation.

Heat and cold can be applied to painful areas of the back in a number of ways. Cold may be applied with a commercially available cold pack that can be placed in your freezer to be frozen and refrozen as needed. You can make your own cold pack by wrapping a towel around a bag of frozen peas or a sealable sandwich bag filled with ice.

Heat may be dry or moist. Dry heat sources include heat lamps or heating pads. Moist heat sources include warm baths and washcloths soaked in warm water.

Before using either hot or cold, be sure your skin is dry and free from cuts and sores. If you have visible skin damage, don't use cold or heat. After using heat or cold, carefully dry the skin and check for purplish-red skin or hives, which may indicate the treatment was too strong. Allow your skin to return to normal temperature and color before using heat or cold again.

For some helpful tips on using heat and cold safely, see "How to Use Hot and Cold" on this page.

How To Use Hot and Cold

Using heat and cold can be an easy and effective way to reduce back pain, inflammation and stiffness that can occur with arthritis or mechanical injury. But like everything, there is a right and wrong way to do it. Follow the suggestions below to get the greatest benefits of your hot and cold treatments and to reduce the risk of harm to the skin and underlying tissue.

- Use heat or cold for only 15 to 20 minutes at a time.
- Avoid using treatments that are extremely hot or cold.
- Always put a towel between your skin and the hot or cold pack.
- Don't use creams, rubs or lotions on your skin with a cold or hot treatment.
- Turn off your heating pad before going to sleep to prevent burns.
- Use an electric blanket or mattress pad. Turn it up before you get out of bed to help ease morning stiffness. Follow the directions on the blanket or pad carefully to ensure safety.
- Use a hot water bottle to keep your back warm.
- Consult your doctor or physical therapist before using cold packs if you have poor circulation, vasculitis or Raynaud's phenomenon, a condition in which blood vessels in the extremities go into spasm – resulting in bluish color and numbness or tingling – in response to cold temperatures or stress.

As with any treatment, follow the advice of your health-care professional when using these methods.

OSTEOPATHY

Osteopathy is a system of medicine that emphasizes body mechanics along with more traditional (*allopathic*) physical, medicinal and surgical methods to diagnose and treat disease.

Osteopathy is performed by osteopathic physicians (DOs), as opposed to medical doctors (MDs). Like MDs, osteopathic physicians complete medical school and training programs and are licensed to prescribe medicine and perform surgery just as MDs are. The main difference is that most osteopathic physicians are trained in manipulative techniques and some DOs' practices focus on hands-on therapy.

The precise therapy you get from an osteopathic physician will be unique, depending on his or her assessment of your pain problem and its cause, but techniques frequently employed are designed to stretch tight muscles and align misplaced bones. Some DOs are trained to provide such therapies as massage, trigger point injections (see Chapter 4) and craniosacral therapy.

ULTRASOUND

Physical therapists often use ultrasound to administer soothing heat to painful tissues. Unlike the superficial heating you get with a heating pad or hot water bottle, the heat created through ultrasound – high-frequency, inaudible sound waves that the body absorbs – goes deep within the tissues.

As with the heat created by more superficial sources, however, the relief ultrasound provides is temporary. If you were to rely solely on ultrasound for relief, you would have to return for treatments frequently.

Ultrasound requires special equipment and must be administered by a health-care professional trained to use it. For that reason, repeated treatments can be impractical and expensive. Doctors are most likely to prescribe it for temporary or occasional use when back pain is particularly severe or when back pain makes activity difficult and/or when you are waiting for other pain treatments to take effect. Ultrasound therapy is not recommended for acute back pain or for pain accompanied by inflammation, because the heat may actually make inflammation worse.

BRACES AND CORSETS

Many people with back pain may benefit from a brace or corset at some point during the course of treatment for back pain. Braces and corsets (elasticized, close-fitting undergarments that support and shape the hips, lower back and abdomen) are typically worn under your clothing and are available in several types.

Corsets are adjustable and made of elastic; braces are sturdier and have metal stays. Both are used for the same purposes: to reduce pressure on the discs, provide back and abdominal support, and stabilize and restrict movement of the back during healing.

Braces are often prescribed for temporary pain relief, especially during times you'll be particularly active or sitting for long periods of time. They often are prescribed for short-term use during recovery from a fractured vertebra or some spine surgeries. For people with certain conditions, including spondylolisthesis or scoliosis, braces may be prescribed longer-term to support the back and restrict movement.

TRANSCUTANEOUS ELECTRICAL NERVE STIMULATION (TENS)

If your pain is severe and doesn't respond to medication or other non-medication therapies, you may be a candidate for **transcutaneous electrical nerve stimulation** (TENS). As its name suggests, TENS is a technique that uses electrical stimulation to the nerves to block pain signals to the brain.

TENS is essentially the same as spinal cord stimulation, which is discussed in Chapter 4, except that instead of implanting electrodes between your vertebrae, your doctor places them on your skin near the painful area. The electrodes are attached to a small battery-operated box (which remains external as well) that emits low-level electrical energy. When the box emits its energy, you receive a low-level shock that will give a tingling sensation, and if all goes well, some temporary relief from your pain.

TENS is not for everyone. Some people will find that their pain does not respond to the treatment; furthermore, it's expensive and it's not appropriate for widespread pain. But for some people with back pain, TENS may provide at least temporary relief when it seems nothing else will.

chapter 7:

The Importance of A Healthy Lifestyle

The best advice for having a healthy, pain-free back doesn't always focus on what to do after back pain has lingered or even started. Often, back pain can be prevented or at least lessened through healthy lifestyle habits – a healthy diet, proper posture, the right footwear choice and, of course, plenty of physical activity. When back pain does occur, these same good habits can ease pain and make its return less likely. In this chapter, we'll discuss some of the lifestyle issues you should address whether you have had ongoing or recurring back pain for some time or if you would just like to lessen your chances of having it.

Exercise

One of the best things you can do for yourself, whether you have health problems or are healthy and want to stay that way, is to exercise. A regular and varied exercise program can ease pain and stiffness, strengthen muscles and bones, burn calories, improve flexibility, increase energy, improve sleep, boost your mood, increase your sense of well-being and reduce your risk of cardiovascular disease and certain cancers.

If your back is so stiff or painful that you can hardly imagine exercising, speak to your doctor or physical therapist about exercises that might be appropriate for you. Then start slowly, set small goals and build from there.

If time, expense or lack of physical conditioning are issues, take heart. Exercise can be worked into your daily schedule in small increments, and it doesn't require membership in an expensive health club. Simply walking around the block – or through the parking deck to your office – or working in your garden can help build muscle strength and endurance, and keep your body moving.

As you become more serious about exercising, however, you may want to add new components to your routine. A well-rounded exercise program should contain three types of exercise:

1. Range-of-motion exercises keep your body flexible. They may involve bending, stretching or swaying.
2. Strengthening exercises build up the muscles that support the spine and other structures. Strengthening exercises can be one of the following:

Isometric – exercises in which a force is applied to a resistant object. An example would be placing both palms together, upright, in front of you (as if you were praying) and pressing them against each other. Isometric exercises can be helpful in strengthening muscles of the back and abdomen that support the spine.

Isotonic – exercise that involves moving a constant, heavy weight through a full range of possible movement. Lifting free weights is an example of isotonic exercise.

Isokinetic – exercise in which the maximum force of which the muscle is capable may be applied through range of motion. Exercise with a Nautilus™ machine is an example of isokinetic exercise.

3. Aerobic or endurance exercises involve sustained use of large muscles and increase the heart rate to strengthen your heart and lungs. Aerobic exercise includes dancing, walking, swimming, jogging and using various exercise machines.

If you have back problems, there are certain exercises to focus on to strengthen the muscles in your abdomen and back that support your spine. Depending on your particular problem, there may be exercises you'll need to avoid. For example, if you have suffered or are at risk for compression fractures of the vertebrae, avoid any high-impact exercises or exercise likely to result in an injury, because when bones are fragile, it doesn't take a lot to make them break (better safe than sorry). Such activities include:

- Jogging
- High-impact aerobics
- Step aerobics
- Football
- Sky diving
- In-line skating
- Snow skiing

Below, we'll describe some exercises you might want to try.

EXERCISE IN WATER

Whether it's in a heated pool at the local YMCA or in the privacy of their own bathtubs or hot tubs, many people with back pain benefit from exercising in water. Exercising in warm water offers several benefits including the following:

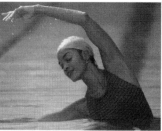

- Warm water allows your muscles to become relaxed, which can make exercise easier. Relaxed muscles can also create an overall feeling of comfort.
- The buoyancy of water makes it possible to exercise in ways that you can't on land. If your spine is fragile due to arthritis, surgery or osteoporotic fractures, water adds comforting support and minimizes the risk of injury that is more likely with land-based exercises.
- Water may act as a force of resistance to help build muscle strength during exercise.

If you'd like to give water exercise a try, contact your local Arthritis Foundation chapter and inquire about the Arthritis Foundation Aquatics Program (AFAP), a water exercise program designed for people with arthritis and related conditions, including back pain. This course could help you increase your strength, flexibility and fitness, so you can better control your back pain.

Classes are usually 45 to 60 minutes in length, and are conducted two or three times per week at local indoor pools. Although AFAP (also held at YMCAs in some areas, where the program is known as AFYAP – Arthritis Foundation YMCA Aquatics Program) will not replace a regimen of therapeutic exercises prescribed by a physician or physical therapist, participants report physical benefits such as decreased pain and stiffness after taking part in the classes. To find the Arthritis Foundation office that serves your area, call 800-283-7800 or log on to www.arthritis.org to request a free copy of "Water Exercise: Pools, Spas and Arthritis."

The following exercises are some you can try in a heated pool, bathtub or hot tub. To learn more exercises you can do in water, consult a physical therapist.

In a Pool:

The following exercises should be done in chest-high water:

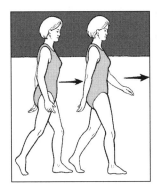

Water walking:

Walk normally across the pool or in a circle. Swing your arms as you walk.

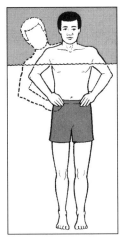

Side bend:

Place your hands on your hips with your feet shoulder-width apart and knees relaxed. Without moving your feet, slowly bend to the right. Return to starting position and bend to the left. Do not bend forward, or twist or turn your trunk. You also may do the exercise with your arms hanging at your sides, with your hand sliding down your thigh as you bend. Repeat the exercise on your left side.

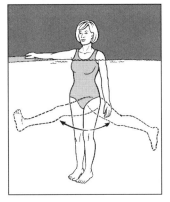

Leg kicks:

Stand at one side of the pool, facing the front of the pool. Hold onto the side with your arm closest to the wall extended. Now, raise the opposite leg as far forward as is comfortable, then bring your leg back down and extend it behind you as far as you comfortably can. Repeat the process several times, then turn and do the same exercise with the opposite leg.

In a Hot Tub:

If you have pain in your upper spine or shoulders, one of the following exercises may help. To perform these exercises, you should be seated in water that reaches approximately to shoulder level:

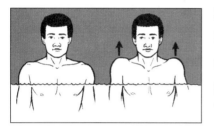

Shoulder shrugs:

Raise your shoulders slowly as if you are shrugging. Hold them in a shrugging position for about 10 seconds. Then, push them back down as far as you can and hold for 10 seconds. Repeat.

Forward arm stretch:

With both arms, reach straight in front of you. Raise your hands overhead as high as possible, keeping your elbows as straight as you can.

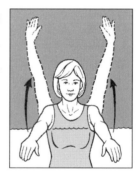

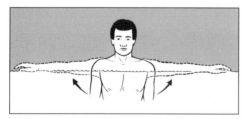

Sideways arm reach:

Slowly raise arms out to the side, keeping your palms down. Raise only to shoulder (water) level. Then lower arms. Do not shrug your shoulders or twist your trunk.

EXERCISE ON LAND

Despite all the benefits of exercising in water, confining your exercise program to a tub or pool isn't always practical or even desirable. Part of exercising is getting out and enjoying the fresh air, seeing new sights and even accomplishing something in the process. In addition, weight-bearing exercise (that is, exercise in which the weight of the body is borne by the large bones of the legs) done on land helps strengthen bones and ward off osteoporosis, thereby reducing your risk of painful vertebral fractures.

Following are some exercises that can strengthen muscles and ease back pain. Before doing any of these exercises, first consult your doctor or physical therapist. A physical therapist may also be able to recommend exercises tailored to your specific condition.

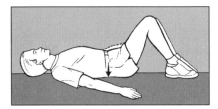

Pelvic Tilts

Lie on your back with knees bent and feet flat on the floor. Tighten your buttocks and roll your pelvis up to flatten your back against the floor. Hold for 15 to 20 seconds. Relax and repeat.

Crunches

Lie with knees bent, arms at your side. Reach for your knees, raising your head and shoulders off the floor. Continue to breathe. Relax to initial position.

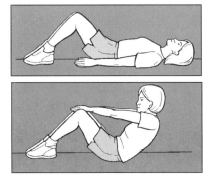

Double Knee Pull

Lie on your back with both knees bent, feet flat. Bring one knee up, then the other, pulling both to your chest until you feel a stretching in your buttocks. Bring your forehead to your knees and hold for 10 seconds. Put one foot down, then the other. Rest and repeat.

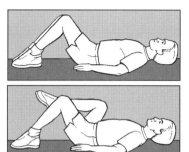

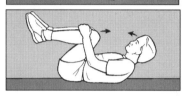

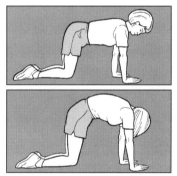

Angry Cat Stretch*

Kneel on your hands and knees. Arch your back up like an angry cat. Hold for 10 seconds. Relax and repeat.

*CAUTION: Do not do this exercise if you have been diagnosed with a ruptured disc.

Seated Toe Touches

Sit in a chair with your feet flat on the floor. Slowly bend toward the floor and reach for your toes (you don't have to touch them). Hold this position for 15 to 30 seconds then slowly rise back up to your original position. Repeat.

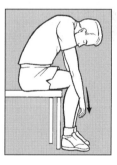

The Benefits of Rest

As beneficial as exercise is, it shouldn't be taken to the extreme. Exercising too much too soon can lead to injury and increased pain. Every one needs time to rest and recuperate.

Bed rest, perhaps, is the most common treatment for back pain. But rest, too, should be done in moderation. If you have an acute flare of pain, stay in bed no longer than a few days. Spending too much time in bed can lead to muscle atrophy, which can make it more difficult for muscles to support the spine. The possible result: Your back pain can worsen.

Back-Healthy Habits

Sometimes the most effective way to ease back pain or prevent its return is to give up old habits and adopt healthy new ones. Everyday patterns and habits, such as slouching, overeating, smoking or sleeping on an old, sagging mattress can add up to create and perpetuate pain.

If you're having back problems, you may need to address the following areas:

POSTURE

"Don't slouch! Sit up straight." It turns out that your mother's advice was well worth heeding. Poor habits such as slouching, hunching over a desk or even pushing your shoulders back too far with your buttocks protruding (known as swayback) can put tension on the spine and lead to back pain.

To see if you have proper posture, try these two simple tests:

Standing or Seated: Stand with a full-length mirror to your side so that when you turn your head you can see your profile. Now, imagine that you have dropped a weighted string from the top of your head to the soles of your feet. Look in the mirror and imagine where the string would fall. If you are standing properly, it should pass through your earlobe, the front of your shoulder, the center of your hip, behind your kneecap and in front of your anklebone.

Now, pull up a chair and have a seat. Imagine again the string dropped from your head. It should pass through the same locations.

Walking: Take a look at the soles of your favorite, well-worn walking shoes. Is the wear evenly distributed on the shoe? Excessive wear on either side of the heel indicates a problem with posture. Your doctor or physical therapist may be able to recommend modifications to improve your posture. Following are some other tests and methods to change your posture.

Improving Your Posture

If those tests reveal your posture isn't perfect, it's time to make changes. By following the same exercise to examine your posture standing or seated, you can train yourself to have better posture. Just practice standing in a way that would make the imaginary string pass through the spots mentioned. When walking or moving, be mindful of your posture. Here are some techniques you might find helpful for postural improvement:

When Standing:

- Stand with weight equally distributed on both feet.
- Place one foot on a footstool to ease tension in your back.
- Wear flat or low-heeled shoes if you stand for long periods of time.
- Keep your back straight by tightening your stomach muscles and buttocks and doing a pelvic tilt.

When Sitting:

- Keep stomach muscles pulled in, and maintain the proper curve in your lower back. You can do this by tightening your stomach and buttocks. Placing a small cushion behind your lower back can help maintain the natural curve of the back.

- Keep your knees slightly higher than your hips. Use a footstool or book under your feet if necessary.
- Don't sit for long periods of time. Stand up and move around periodically to stretch tight muscles and give them a chance to relax.

LIFTING METHODS

What do you do when you have a heavy box or a small (or not-so-small) child to lift? Your answer can make a big difference in your back health. To prevent back injuries or to keep old injuries from recurring, follow these tips for lifting or carrying:

- Face your work when lifting or carrying objects.
- Bend and lift using your knees and legs instead of your back.
- Hold the object close to you.
- Straighten your legs to lift the object.
- Get help to lift objects that are too heavy.

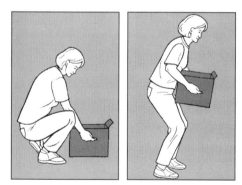

CORRECT

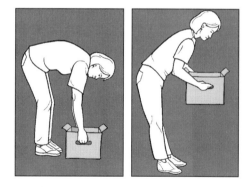

INCORRECT

SLEEPING

If you awaken often with a backache*, it may be time to evaluate your sleeping habits and your mattress. Most people find it most comfortable to sleep on a firm, but not too firm, mattress. Try placing a piece of plywood (approximately $3/4$-inch thick) under a soft mattress to provide firmness.

If you normally sleep on your stomach, make every effort to fall asleep on your side or back. If you awaken in the night on your stomach, roll over. Sleeping on your stomach provides the least support for your spine.

When going to sleep on your back, try placing a pillow under your knees. When going to sleep on your side, try to keep your legs bent at the knees and the hips.

If pain makes it difficult to fall asleep or stay asleep, or if lack of sleep contributes to your pain, speak to your doctor about the possibility of prescribing medications that relieve pain and aid sleep. For general tips on how to get a better night's sleep, see "Tips for a Good Night's Sleep" on the next page.

* NOTE: If you frequently awaken with back pain that goes away after urination, you may have a problem called vesicoureteral reflux, in which the urine from the bladder flows back up into the ureters (the two thin tubes that carry urine from the kidneys to the bladder). Because the condition can lead to more serious urinary tract problems if not treated, it's important to consult your primary-care physician, who may need to refer you to a urologist (a doctor who specializes in treating conditions of the urinary tract).

Tips for a Good Night's Sleep

If you often wake up unrefreshed, or if fatigue is contributing to your pain, try the following tips to help improve your sleep. If you still have trouble sleeping, speak to your doctor about the possibility of medication.

- **Pick a time to go to bed and get up every day.** Stick with your schedule.

- **Avoid naps, if possible.** If you feel you must nap, set an alarm to go off 30 minutes later. Avoid napping in the afternoon or evening.

- **Steer clear of caffeinated foods and beverages, particularly in the afternoon and evening.** Caffeine can be found in soft drinks (even the yellow-colored ones), colas, tea, coffee, chocolate and even some over-the-counter pain relievers. (Be sure to check labels!)

- **Be sure to get regular exercise.** Nothing promotes a good night's sleep like exercise, but you may want to experiment by exercising at different times of the day to see which works best. Some people find that exercising within a few hours of bedtime keeps them awake.

- **Stop smoking.** Nicotine, like caffeine, is a stimulant. Besides, there are plenty of other reasons to stop smoking.

- **Try a warm bath before bedtime.** Some people find the warm water relaxes muscles, making it easier to sleep, but others find it invigorating.

- **Limit bedtime distractions.** Keep your bedroom dark, cool and quiet. Reserve your bed for sleeping and sex. That means no newspapers, briefcases, suspense novels or TV.

- **Get up if you can't sleep.** Stay in bed for about half an hour. If sleep eludes you, get up and do something boring (like reading the telephone white pages) for 30 minutes, and then try again to sleep.

DIET AND WEIGHT MANAGEMENT

There's not much worse for your back than being overweight. Excess pounds shift your center of gravity forward, creating added stress on your lower back. If you are overweight and have back pain, losing weight may significantly ease the problem.

The secret to weight loss is really no secret: You must burn more calories than you consume. For most people that means increasing your level of exercise, while decreasing the amount you eat.

For optimal health – whether you have arthritis or not – it's important to consume a healthful diet that is rich in vitamins and minerals, low in saturated fats, and sensible in calories. The proper diet can also reduce your risk of hypertension and high cholesterol, two health conditions that recently have been linked to back pain.

Sample Diets To Follow

Most doctors advise their patients to follow a diet such as those recommended by the American Heart Association (online at www.americanheart.org) or American Cancer Society (on the Web at www.cancer.org), both of which emphasize fruits, vegetables and grains.

Another good general guideline for a balanced daily food intake is the USDA's Food Guide Pyramid, a visual diagram of the government agency's recommended healthy diet. The foods at the base of the pyramid should make up the bulk of your diet, the foods in the middle should be eaten in moderate quantities, and the foods at the very top of the pyramid should be eaten sparingly. The suggested diet emphasizes building your daily food intake on a base of low-fat, high-fiber breads, grains and complex carbohydrates; eating several servings a day of fruits and vegetables; including moderate amounts of lean proteins, such as fish, meats and poultry; eating moderate servings of dairy products, which add calcium; and eating small amounts of fats, sugars and oils.

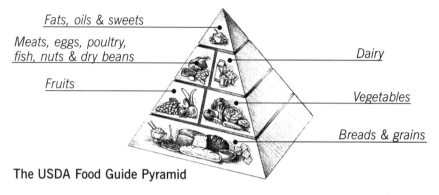

Fats, oils & sweets

Meats, eggs, poultry, fish, nuts & dry beans

Fruits

Dairy

Vegetables

Breads & grains

The USDA Food Guide Pyramid

Special Considerations

Some people have special situations that may benefit from extra doses of certain nutrients. For example, if you have osteoporosis or risk factors for it, consuming plenty of calcium-rich products, including fortified juices and low-fat dairy products, is important for strong bones. (See "Osteoporosis Risk Factors" page 10.)

If you are between the ages of 19 and 50, you need 1,000 milligrams (mg) of calcium per day. If you're 51 or older, you need 1,200 mg daily. Your doctor may recommend higher doses if you have established osteoporosis. For good food sources of calcium, along with their calcium content, see "Food Sources of Calcium" on page 123.

In addition, people with inflammatory problems, including rheumatoid arthritis that affects the spine or ankylosing spondylitis, may benefit from changing the types of fats and oils in their diets. Oils such as safflower, sunflower and corn, as well as the fats in meat and poultry, may contribute to inflammation, whereas olive, canola and flaxseed oils and fats in cold-water fish may help to reduce inflammation.

If you are concerned about your weight and need help finding a diet that you can stick with, consult your physician or a registered dietitian.

Food Sources of Calcium

If you're concerned about the amount of calcium you're consuming, try to eat plenty of your favorites from the following:

Food	Serving Size	Calcium content (in milligrams)
Baked beans	1 cup	163
Brazil nuts	$1/2$ cup	130
Broccoli (cooked, fresh)	1 cup	136
Cheddar cheese	1 ounce	204
Macaroni and cheese	$1/2$ cup	180 (approximately)
Milk (whole, 2% or skim)	1 cup	300
Salmon, canned with bones	$3\,3/4$ -ounce can	225
Spinach, cooked	$1/2$ cup	300
Yogurt, plain	1 cup	415

FOOTWEAR

Sometimes easing back pain is as simple as wearing the right shoes, particularly if you spend a lot of time standing or walking. Wearing shoes with high heels or heels with uneven wear, for example, can throw off your posture and, in turn, place unnecessary stress on your back. When choosing shoes, look for the following:

A durable counter (the part of the shoe that surrounds your heel). A shoe that allows your heel to move inward or outward can create stress on your lower back.

A supportive insole. The insole should cushion your heel and support your arch.

A roomy toe box (the area of the shoe that houses your toes). It should allow your toes to move comfortably while supporting the sides of your feet.

A flexible sole. A sole that doesn't bend at the ball of your foot is uncomfortable and throws off your posture by causing you to walk in an awkward manner.

A padded heel. The heel should absorb shock as you walk. It should not be too narrow or too wide; it should be the same width as the heel counter.

TOBACCO USE

If you haven't heard enough reasons over the years to make you want to stop smoking, here's another: Cigarette smoke is bad for your back. Recent research has shown a high prevalence of spinal stenosis and back pain among smokers. One suspected reason is that smoking causes damage to blood vessels that supply the back.

In addition to that, cigarette smoke is bad for your bones. Smoking is a risk factor for osteoporosis, which can lead to painful vertebral fractures. If you smoke and need back surgery, there's more bad news. Smoking can interfere with healing, and spinal fusions performed in smokers are significantly more likely to fail than the same surgery in nonsmokers.

STRESS REDUCTION

Regardless of the problem – injury, disease or something else – that initiated your back pain, one of the biggest factors in the persistence of pain and its effects on your daily life is stress. Let's face it: Being in pain is stressful, and being under stress can add to your pain.

Because stress and pain go hand in hand, there is not a clear line between stress-reduction therapies and pain-reduction therapies. However, we have attempted to draw a line for the purposes of this book. Anything you do to ease pain will help ease stress and anything you do to ease stress has the potential to ease your pain.

Although for this chapter we chose methods used primarily for pain relief, some of these methods may help relieve stress. For example, you may have – or give yourself – a massage as a way to ease pain and relax. Similarly you may take a walk – or a yoga class – or soak in a warm tub to relieve stress and pain.

In Chapter 8, we'll discuss some activities and techniques you may pursue purely for relaxation. Don't be surprised if they have the pleasant side effect of easing your pain as well! Right now, let's look at some other, less traditional ways to relieve your back pain.

chapter 8

Another Way: Complementary and Alternative Therapies

If your back is in constant pain, it's only natural that you would be willing to try just about anything to make the pain go away. That's why, each year, millions of Americans – and their numbers are growing – try alternative therapies.

Also referred to as complementary therapies or, sometimes, "unproven" remedies, alternative therapies usually are defined as those for which there is little, if any, scientific research to back their use. Unlike prescription and over-the-counter medications, alternative therapies have not undergone the rigorous scientific review that is required for drugs to receive FDA approvals.

Many of these therapies were used frequently by practitioners not so many years ago. As modern medicines and surgical techniques were developed, however, most Western doctors abandoned traditional remedies for scientifically proven therapies.

But for some alternative therapies, everything old is new again. Now modern medicine is the "traditional" approach and age-old remedies seem like a fresh approach.

As many treatments once again start to gain acceptance among patients and physicians, they are being put to the test scientifically. In the late 1990s, the federal government formed the National Center for Complementary and Alternative Medicine (NCCAM) at the National Institutes of Health (NIH) to conduct and support clinical and basic research into complementary and alternative therapies. One of the largest areas of supported research focuses on alternative therapies for musculoskeletal problems.

Interestingly, pain problems – which often involve the musculoskeletal system – are among the most common reasons people try alternative therapies. Symptoms like pain and stiffness also are among those most likely to be helped by alternative therapies. Why? Scientists suspect the reason is that such symptoms are subjective (that is, there is no way to objectively measure them, as you would measure body temperature, for example). Another reason may be the **placebo effect**. The placebo effect is a phenomenon where a person feels an improvement in symptoms although he or she has taken an inert, or useless, substance (such as a sugar pill). The relief occurs for the simple reason that the person believes the therapy will work.

Until scientists better understand the various alternative therapies and how they do or don't work, it pays to proceed with caution as you explore such treatments. Although many alternative therapies are considered natural, remember that many "natural" things – arsenic, uranium and poison ivy, to name a few – are toxic, meaning they could damage your health. As one scientist said, "Anything with the strength to do good also has the strength to do harm."

If you are interested in trying an alternative therapy, first speak with your doctor and be sure to alert him or her to what you're planning to try, particularly if you are taking prescription or over-the-counter medications. Products such as nutritional supplements may interact with your medications, either adding to or interfering with their action. Perhaps more dangerous is the possibility that by choosing to use alternatives on your own, you may neglect getting proper treatment for a problem that requires medication or surgery.

In this chapter, we'll take a look at some alternative or complementary therapies used or promoted for back pain.

Nutritional Supplements

As consumers become more aware of the role of nutrition in disease, and as many people become interested in returning to "natural" medicine – particularly for problems that conventional medicine has failed to relieve completely – the manufacture and sale of nutritional supplements is booming.

Nutritional supplements, also called dietary supplements, include herbal remedies as well as vitamins, minerals and enzymes. In the following section, we'll take a closer look at some of the different types of nutritional supplements and some of the specific products touted for back pain.

HERBAL REMEDIES

Long before the advent of modern medicine, doctors used herbs to treat medical conditions as diverse as labor pains and warts. Herbs are plants or parts of plants used for medicines, spices or fragrances. Herbal remedies come in a number of forms, including the following:

- **Whole herbs:** parts of plants that are dried, cut and powdered.
- **Herb teas:** beverages made from steeping herbs in hot or boiling water.

- **Tinctures:** solutions created when an herb is soaked in alcohol or glycerin.
- **Extracts:** tinctures in which some of the alcohol has been distilled out.
- **Capsules and tablets:** herbal preparations made by removing the liquid from an extract, crushing the remaining dry herb into powder form and then filling a capsule or forming a tablet with the powder.
- **Salves and ointments:** topical (rub-on) preparations that contain herbal extracts.

There are more than 100 prescription drugs manufactured from various plants or parts of plants. The term herbal remedy, however, refers to the largely untested, unregulated herbal products you can purchase without a prescription at most any pharmacy or health food store. Again, use caution: An herbal remedy can be very potent. Consult your doctor or pharmacist before taking any herbal remedy.

Following are some of the most common herbal remedies touted for relief of back problems:

Boswellia

Boswellia serrata is a tree from Asia that yields oils, gum and other products when its bark is peeled away. The gum has long been used in Indian Ayurvedic medicine for arthritis and musculoskeletal pain. In animal and test-tube studies, boswellia interferes with the synthesis of inflammation-causing chemicals and, therefore, may have some anti-inflammatory effects.

Cat's Claw

In its native Peruvian Amazon, a wild vine commonly referred to as cat's claw (because of its claw-shaped thorns) has had a long tradition as a treatment for inflammation and "bone pain." A study conducted in recent years suggests that, in fact, cat's claw may have anti-inflammatory properties.

Devil's Claw

This folk remedy from Africa is named for the bumpy hooks that cover its fruit. The roots of the plant contain a substance that has anti-inflammatory and pain-relieving properties. In a 1998 study of 118 patients with chronic low back pain, devil's claw was found to be significantly better than placebo for pain relief.

Ginger

A staple of Asian cooking, ginger may do more than add flavor to foods. Laboratory research shows ginger (a root found in supermarkets) may also have pain-relieving and anti-inflammatory properties.

St. John's Wort

A small, yellow flower that grows throughout Europe and the United States, St. John's wort is one of the top-selling herbal remedies in the United States. One of its most touted benefits is relieving depression, which can be both a result of and contributor to back pain. St. John's wort may also have some anti-inflammatory effects.

VITAMINS

If you eat a varied diet rich in fruits and vegetables, ideally, you should not need vitamin supplements. Yet certain medications and chronic diseases can affect your body's absorption of vitamins or increase your need for certain ones. Most doctors recommend that patients with any potential nutrient deficiencies take a multiple vitamin supplement (such as *One-A-Day* or *Centrum*). Beyond that, other vitamin supplements should be used only to meet particular nutritional needs. Vitamins should never be taken in large doses for curative purposes, because they have potentially dangerous side effects.

Following are some vitamins that may be useful if you have diseases that cause back pain. Ask your doctor about the advisability of taking these or any other vitamins as well as the dose you should take:

Vitamin B3. One study showed it could improve the pain-relieving effects of NSAIDs.

Vitamin C. There is evidence that vitamin C may decrease the risk of progression of OA, which is a common source of back pain.

Vitamin D. Vitamin D is important to strong bones (see "Supplements You Need for Strong Bones," page 135). One study showed that OA progression was higher in people with low vitamin D consumption.

Vitamin E. Research suggests that vitamin E may help ease pain.

MINERALS, ENZYMES AND OTHERS

Nutritional supplements may come from a variety of plant, animal and mineral sources as diverse as bee pollen, cattle cartilage and crab shells. The following non-herbal nutritional supplements are among those most commonly promoted for back health and/or the relief of back pain.

Boron

Boron is a trace mineral that helps our bodies use calcium and magnesium and fights inflammation. There is some evidence that boron can ease symptoms associated with osteoporotic fractures, osteoarthritis and rheumatoid arthritis, all of which can affect the spine.

Bromelain

Bromelain is a protein-digesting enzyme derived from pineapple. Because it may relieve muscle tension, it is sometimes recommended for sprains and strains. There is scientific evidence that bromelain has some anti-inflammatory effect.

Calcium

Calcium is perhaps the most important mineral for strong bones. If you don't get enough calcium in your diet, a supplement is essential. For more about calcium and specific daily requirements, see "Supplements You Need for Strong Bones" on page 135.

Chondroitin Sulfate

Derived from cattle trachea, chondroitin sulfate has been used in Europe for years for osteoarthritis (OA) pain. Since the mid-'90s, it has been used widely in the United States as well. Although it hasn't been proven to reverse cartilage loss, in some studies it did appear to stop joint degeneration. So far, none of these studies have focused on OA found in the spine.

Copper

Copper is a trace mineral that plays a role in bone growth and may help prevent bone loss. Copper may also ease inflammation.

Fish Oil

Oils from cold-water fish, such as salmon or mackerel, show promise for relieving arthritis, which may affect your back. Fish oil contains the omega-3 fatty acids eicosapentaenoic acid (EPA) and docosahexaenoic acid (DHA) that appear to ease arthritis symptoms. Taken cautiously, fish oil supplements may ease back pain and inflammation associated with arthritis.

Glucosamine

Glucosamine is a natural substance that provides the building blocks for the body to make and repair cartilage. Glucosamine supplements are extracted from crab, lobster or shrimp shells. They have been used to treat arthritis in animals for years, but only in the past decade have become popular for use in people with osteoarthritis. Studies show that glucosamine may ease pain as well as nonsteroidal anti-inflam-matory drugs (NSAIDs) do in people with OA of the knee; however, the supplement has not been studied for OA back pain. There is specula-tion – but no scientific evidence, yet – that glucosamine may help rebuild damaged cartilage.

Magnesium

Magnesium is a mineral needed for healthy tissue and bone. Studies suggest magnesium supplements may help ease the pain and fatigue of fibromyalgia, which may affect your back.

SAM (S-adenosylmethionine)

SAM, often called SAM-e (pronounced like "Sammy"), is a naturally occurring compound in the body. Studies of SAM show it relieves osteoarthritis pain about as well as NSAIDs without NSAIDs' side effects. SAM is also reported to be an antidepressant, which may be an important bonus, since pain often causes and is worsened by depression.

✳ BE AWARE:

Unlike prescription and over-the-counter medications, the nutritional supplements and herbal remedies you find in health-food stores and in your grocery store's natural remedies section are not required to undergo the same rigorous process required to obtain Food and Drug Administration approval.

There is no proof an alternative remedy will do anything or is safe. Nor are there any assurances that the package will contain what the label says. In fact, some recent studies by an independent laboratory showed that several products included potentially harmful ingredients that were not listed on the product labels. Many products did not contain the ingredients promised or they contained smaller amounts of ingredients than the labels listed.

If you want to try nutritional supplements, be sure to purchase them from a reputable dealer and look for the words "standard" or "standardized" on the label, which means that the supplement meets an international standard of quality.

Supplements You Need for Strong Bones

If you want to prevent painful fractures of your spine, there are two supplements you should definitely know about: calcium and vitamin D. Calcium, a mineral, is a main component of bones. Vitamin D helps the calcium you consume do its job.

Your body manufactures vitamin D in response to sunlight, but if you live in the northern United States, avoid sun exposure or always wear sunscreen, you may not be making enough. (This does not mean you should run out and soak up the sun's rays unprotected. There are many ways to get vitamin D!) Both calcium and vitamin D are also available in a varied diet, but are sorely lacking in the diets of most Americans – particularly women.

The specific amount of these nutrients that you need varies as you age. For strong bones, doctors and dietitians recommend 1,000 milligrams of calcium daily for adults between the ages of 19 and 50, and 1,200 milligrams daily for those over 50. If you already have osteoporosis, your doctor may advise you to increase your calcium intake. Vitamin D requirements range from 200 international units (IU) to 600 IU per day.

If you aren't getting the optimal amount of either or both nutrients in your diet (see the diet section in Chapter 7 for foods rich in these nutrients), you should consider a supplement. Your doctor or dietitian can help you determine the best supplement and the right daily dosage for you.

When Buying Supplements: Read the Label

To comply with a law that took effect in 1999, nutritional supplement manufacturers are required to put "Supplement Facts" information on their labels, similar to the "Nutritional Facts" panels you have seen on foods for several years now.

Supplement labels must specify active ingredients, with other ingredients in descending order of predominance. Ingredients must be listed by common name along with how much of the supplement you should take in a normal or recommended dose.

Other information required on labels includes the quantity of the container's contents (such as "100 tablets"), directions for use, and the name and location of the manufacturer, packer or distributor (this is the address you should write to for more information). Along with any claim about the product's purported efficacy or application, the label must state, "This statement has not been evaluated by the Food and Drug Administration. This product is not intended to diagnose, treat, cure or prevent any disease."

Movement Therapies

If a bad back makes you cringe at the thought of exercise, a kinder, gentler exercise plan may be just what you need to get you moving again. Here, we'll talk about some alternative forms of exercise that you might want to try. They range from ancient martial arts to 20th-century movement education programs. See if one of these practices appeals to you.

YOGA

Practiced around the world, **yoga** is part of the traditional Indian healing system called Ayurveda. It is one of the oldest known systems of health.

The word yoga means "union." It is the coming together of physical, mental and spiritual energies to enhance well-being. Yoga's breathing exercises, postures and meditation practices, when performed daily, can improve flexibility and balance, regulate heart rate, lower blood pressure, increase muscle strength, and reduce and ease pain, including back pain.

Although there are several branches of yoga practice, the form you're most likely familiar with is hatha yoga. Hatha yoga consists of breathing exercises (*pranayama*) and gentle stretches (*asanas*) that condition the whole body.

If you are interested in trying yoga, many colleges, community centers, senior centers, health clubs and even workplaces offer yoga classes. Before signing up for a yoga class, it's best to speak with your physician.

SAMPLE YOGA EXERCISES:

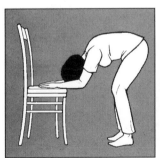 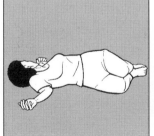 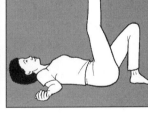

Standing forward bend   *Lying Spinal Twist*   *Single leg raise*

TAI CHI

Although its roots are in martial arts, **tai chi** is not confrontational. It consists of controlled movements that flow rhythmically into one long, graceful gesture. The movement sequences have poetic names such as "white crane spreads its wings" or "part the wild horse's mane."

Research has shown that tai chi improves balance and therefore reduces the risk of falling, which could be serious for a person with fragile bones and joints. Because of its gentle, graceful movements, it's a good form of exercise for people with painful back problems.

The best way to learn tai chi is by taking a course. Many health or community centers, hospitals and schools offer tai chi courses. Courses at each ability level usually last six to eight weeks. After completing a class, you can move to the next ability level. Although traditional tai chi consists of more than 100 movements, most modern classes teach only 24 to 48 positions.

SAMPLE TAI CHI EXERCISES:

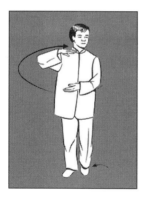

Part the Wild Horse's Mane

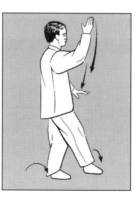

White Crane Spreads Its Wings

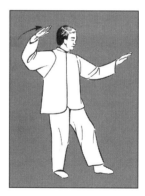

Reverse Reeling Forearm

ALEXANDER TECHNIQUE

Have a seat in a comfortable chair and cross your legs. Now look down. Is your left leg over your right leg, or is your right leg over your left? Now switch, so that the leg you first placed on top is now on the bottom. Does it feel a little weird? Probably. The reason is you're not used to sitting that way.

The order of your legs when you cross them is largely a learned behavior or habit. It is just one of the habits you practice each day without realizing that you do it. In many cases, these patterns of movement – such as the way we bend, reach, walk or even cross our legs – can lead to back pain and other problems.

The **Alexander technique** teaches proper posture through mind-body awareness. It helps you to become aware of habits that may be causing or contributing to pain and then to replace them with healthier ones. The technique has three steps: Be aware of the habit, inhibit your reaction and develop a new mental direction.

The Alexander technique is taught one-on-one, using guiding touch and instruction, in private sessions. Although you may start to see the benefits of improved habits immediately, most instructors recommend as many as 30 sessions.

FELDENKRAIS

Like the Alexander technique, **Feldenkrais** is often taught in private, one-on-one sessions. However, it may be taught in classes.

The Feldenkrais method uses a program of subtle movement to help you become more aware of your body, discover how your body moves and explore new movement skills. The method consists of more than a thousand different movements designed to increase body awareness, flexibility and range of motion. Feldenkrais practitioners use a combination of these movements, along with hands-on manipulations, to gradually teach the body to work more efficiently.

Feldenkrais movements are usually done while you are lying on a floor mat. A private session followed by a six-week series of classes is recommended.

PILATES

The **Pilates** (pronounced pill-AH-tees) method is a system of conditioning that emphasizes proper body alignment, injury prevention and proper breathing techniques. The Pilates method was developed in the 1920s, and has gained widespread popularity in recent years. While other movement therapies may focus on various parts of the body or on the body as a whole, Pilates focuses on the role of the back and spine in health. Through muscle strengthening and stretching exercises, Pilates attempts to develop your lower back and abdomen into a firm core of support for your whole body. It also promotes alignment and stabilization of the spine.

Pilates movements are performed on a bench-like piece of exercise equipment. Pilates training is usually conducted in one-on-one sessions or in small groups.

✳ **BE AWARE:**

While most movement therapies are safe for most people, it's always important to inform your instructor or trainer of back pain and any health problems. There may be some moves you can't do. Also, because many of these methods are taught one on one, they can be an expensive proposition. Insurance doesn't always cover them.

Whichever therapy you choose, it's important to find an instructor experienced in your particular problem. Once you have learned the moves through a qualified instructor, some therapies – for example, yoga or tai chi – may be practiced with an instructional videotape. Your instructor or physical therapist may be able to recommend a videotape that's appropriate for people with your particular problem.

Relaxation Therapies and Techniques

One of the most common contributors to back pain in our society is probably stress. Stress causes muscles to tense, leading to pain. Stress can turn minor pains into bigger pains and can leave you so frazzled that you hardly feel like dealing with pain.

For all of these reasons, relaxation techniques and therapies can be effective in easing both pain itself and pain's effect on your daily life. Popular techniques that have helped people with back pain include visualization, self-hypnosis, meditation and deep breathing. All of these techniques and more are discussed in Chapter 9, "Managing Stress."

ACUPUNCTURE AND ACUPRESSURE

The ancient Asian practice of **acupuncture** and its needle-free varia-tion, **acupressure**, have gained acceptance in the Western world in recent years, particularly for relieving pain.

Acupuncture

A key component of Chinese traditional medicine, acupuncture is based on the theory that essential life energy called qi (pronounced "chee") flows through the body along invisible channels called meridians that touch every organ. According to this theory, illness can unbalance your qi, and out-of-balance qi can cause illness or pain. Stimulation of specific points (called acupoints), where meridians reach the skin surface, can help correct the flow of qi to optimize health or block pain.

In the most familiar form of acupuncture in this country, fine needles are inserted into acupoints to manipulate qi. Sometimes the needles are connected to a low-level electrical current (electroacupuncture) for a more powerful effect. Other forms of acupuncture use heat, herbs, magnets and even bee stings to manipulate qi.

The specific acupoints stimulated differ, depending on the particular problem being treated, and the points aren't necessarily in locations where you might suspect. Back pain, for example, may be treated by stimulating points in your feet.

Although modern scientists don't subscribe to the qi theory, acupuncture may be an effective pain reliever for some people. The best explanation as to how it works: Stimulating acupoints in turn stimulates the nervous system to release the natural pain-killing substances called endorphins and possibly other chemicals that carry messages between nerve cells. This stimulation changes the experience of pain.

Acupuncture is performed by a practitioner called an acupuncturist. Many, but not all, states require acupuncturists to be licensed. Most of this country's estimated 10,000 acupuncturists are not medical doctors; however, an estimated 4,000 U.S. doctors do have some type of acupuncture training.

Before undergoing acupuncture, let your acupuncturist know if you have any health conditions other than the pain being treated. Also, be sure he or she uses sterilized or disposable needles.

Acupressure

Much like acupuncture, acupressure is a technique that, according to ancient beliefs, restores the flow of energy that moves through the body. And like acupuncture, acupressure focuses on stimulation of specific acupoints. Instead of stimulating points with needles, electricity or heat, however, acupressure relies on simple pressure, usually performed with the hands.

Because acupressure is non-invasive and doesn't require a trained professional to administer it, it is a therapy you can experiment with on your own at home. It's best, however, to first take a quick course from someone knowledgeable about the therapy to get optimal benefits.

MAGNETIC THERAPY

Read enough health magazines or visit enough natural health stores and you're bound to hear plenty of claims about the healing benefits of magnets. And you'll probably find many magnet products – ranging from belts and bracelets to mattress pads – designed to ease your pain and other ailments.

Although magnets have been touted as pain-relievers for years, only recently have a few scientific studies suggested that they may actually have some benefits against pain. No one knows exactly how magnets might work (or if they really do), but some experts suspect they increase blood flow to the painful area. Increased blood flow carries oxygen to the injured area, decreasing inflammation, relieving pain and, perhaps, promoting healing. Another possible explanation is that magnets disrupt pain signals going to the brain.

In magnetic therapy, certain parts of the body are exposed to magnet fields. For back pain, this most likely means placing magnets at various locations on the back, wearing a belt with magnets in it or sleeping on a magnetic mattress pad.

✳ BE AWARE:

Although it's probably safe to use magnets in most circumstances, there's little reason to believe they will help. You should never use a magnet close to an implanted device such as a pacemaker. If you are pregnant, avoid using magnets on your abdomen.

HANDS-ON THERAPIES

Some of the most soothing therapies for back pain rely on human touch. Here are some widely (and some not-so-widely) used hands-on therapies for back pain.

Chiropractic

Each year, as many as 40 percent of people who experience back pain visit a **chiropractor** for it. Chiropractors are practitioners who are trained and licensed to practice **chiropractic**, a therapy that, depending on the chiropractor's training, may focus on the manual adjustment of the spine.

The term and the therapy were created in Davenport, Iowa, in 1895 by a charismatic entrepreneur named Daniel David Palmer. Palmer founded chiropractic based on the theory that misalignment of vertebrae, called subluxation, is the cause of almost all diseases, and chiropractic adjustment of the spine is the cure. Today, not all chiropractors subscribe to the belief that spinal adjustment can cure anything; many focus on relieving musculoskeletal problems.

Chiropractic adjustment involves manipulating the areas of the spine that correspond to the location of the pain, thus relieving irritating pressure on the vertebrae and nerves. The specific treatment and number of treatments you'll receive from a chiropractor will depend on his or her assessment of your problem through a physical exam and imaging tests (see section on diagnostic tests on page 23) such as X-rays and, sometimes, blood tests.

✳ BE AWARE:

While chiropractic adjustment generally is safe, even most chiropractors agree that there are cases when back pain requires more than chiropractic. If you have a severe back problem or disease that doesn't respond to chiropractic or seems to be beyond the chiropractor's scope of expertise, it's important that you see a medical doctor or surgeon.

Reflexology

Instead of focusing on the acupoints along meridians as acupressure and acupuncture do, **reflexology** supposedly works by stimulating nerve endings in the ears, hands and feet.

Because reflexology is completely non-invasive and you don't have to be able to reach your back to do it, reflexology is a good therapy to try on your own. It can't hurt, and it might help. On page 146, you'll find the charts that reflexologists use to identify nerve endings that correspond with specific areas of the spine. For example, if you have pain in your lower back, you would need to stimulate nerve endings between the palm and wrist. Stimulating nerve endings approximately a half-inch below that would ease sciatic pain. For neck pain, you could stimulate nerve endings on the outer side of your big toe or the area between your little toe and the one next to it.

To try reflexology, find a place where you will be undisturbed for 10 to 15 minutes. When doing foot reflexology, remove your shoes and socks and rub your feet with lotion. Apply gentle pressure – with your fingers or a blunt, soft object such as a pencil eraser – to the appropriate spots and then release. You can tell better than anyone can how much pressure is required to get results.

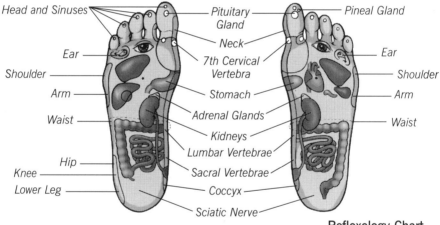

Head and Sinuses — Pituitary Gland — Pineal Gland
Ear — Neck — Ear
Shoulder — 7th Cervical Vertebra — Shoulder
Arm — Stomach — Arm
Waist — Adrenal Glands — Waist
Kidneys
Lumbar Vertebrae
Hip — Sacral Vertebrae
Knee — Coccyx
Lower Leg — Sciatic Nerve

Refloxology Chart

Myotherapy

A hands-on treatment, **myotherapy** involves applying pressure to trigger points – points on the body that, when pressed, cause pain at another location in the body (or refer readers to previous reference to trigger points) – using the fingers, knuckles and elbows. Although no one knows precisely how myotherapy works, many people say it relieves their pain.

Back pain is the number one reason why people have myotherapy.

Myotherapy is typically performed by a certified myotherapist; however, after a few visits with and instruction from a myotherapist, you can probably train a friend or partner to perform myotherapy that targets your trigger points.

The Benefits of Alternatives

If you feel frustrated by back pain that just won't go away with conventional therapy, alternative and complementary therapies – when used wisely – may offer benefits in addition to the those you get from your doctor-prescribed medication alone. These therapies also may give you the satisfaction that you are doing something for your problem. Some of these remedies eventually may be scientifically proven to do what they claim.

Should you decide to proceed with an alternative or complementary therapy, it's important to understand as much as you can about the therapy. This book can serve as a starting point, but it is just that – a starting point. For some helpful advice on making the decision about alternatives, see "Evaluating Alternative and Complementary Therapies" on page 148. It's also important not to abandon any proven therapies that your doctor prescribes, particularly if your pain is caused by a disease that can progress if not treated. You should discuss any alternative therapy with your doctor. You and your doctor should work together to make a decision about whether or not to try it.

One alternative therapy, which we have discussed only briefly in this chapter, is stress management and relaxation. If your back pain leaves you feeling powerless, learning stress-management techniques can empower you. While you can't always change the stressors in your life, the way react to them is entirely up to you. In the following chapter, we'll show you how to learn new ways to react more positively – and healthfully, for your back – to stress.

Evaluating Alternative and Complementary Therapies

When you're considering a complementary or alternative therapy, it pays to be cautious. In your search for relief, you may be willing to try something that helps nothing but the wallet of the person selling it. Never assume a product is safe just because it's natural.

Follow this advice if you think you might like to try an alternative or complementary therapy:

Know the facts. Although drugs and other conventional therapies are monitored and regulated by government agencies like the FDA, such therapies as herbs, supplements and some other alternatives do not have to undergo that type of scrutiny to be marketed.

Use good judgment. If a practitioner makes unrealistic claims such as, "It will cure your back pain," or suggests you discontinue your conventional treatments, consider it a strong warning that something is not right.

Seek out information. A good source of information is the National Center for Complementary and Alternative Medicine (NCCAM). For a free packet of information on alternative therapies, write to the NCCAM Clearinghouse, P.O. Box 8218, Silver Spring, MD 20807-8218. For accurate and easy-to-understand information about alternatives for arthritis-related conditions, check out the Arthritis Foundation's Guide to Alternative Therapies. It's available at bookstores or by calling 800/207-8633 or logging on to www.arthritis.org.

Be a skeptic. Beware of treatments that claim to work by a secret formula, say they are a cure or miraculous breakthrough, or are publicized in the backs of magazines, over the phone or through direct mail. Bona fide treatments are reported in medical journals. Beware of any product that relies on testimonials as proof that it works.

Discuss it with your doctor. Your doctor should be informed about any therapy you're trying, whether or not it is an alternative remedy. He or she can help you watch for and safeguard against side effects and possible negative interactions with medications you may be taking. Your doctor may be able to answer important questions, such as how the therapy fits into your treatment plan and what precautions you should take.

Consider the cost. Some alternative therapies can be costly and most aren't covered by your health insurance. Read your policy closely to find what therapies are covered and under what circumstances these therapies are covered. Then compare your ultimate cost of an alternative to that of a doctor-prescribed medication or treatment.

Proceed with caution. If you decide to go through with an alternative treatment, seek out a qualified practitioner. A state or national board must license practitioners of certain therapies. If that isn't the case for the therapy you're considering, find out about professional societies that provide certification.

Don't abandon a treatment that works. When starting an alternative therapy, don't stop taking the medication your doctor prescribes. Doing so could set you up for additional problems.

chapter 9

Managing Stress: The Beast That Can Hurt Your Back

There's probably not a person alive who doesn't live with some stress. Most of us deal with stresses – work deadlines, traffic jams, demanding bosses or spouses, uncooperative children, appliances or automobiles that break down, roofs that leak, bills that mount (you get the picture) – on a daily basis.

When you feel stressed, your muscles become tense. Muscle tension can, in turn, increase your pain and may limit your abilities, which can lead to depression. A vicious cycle of stress, pain, limited/lost abilities and depression may develop.

If you have back pain, you're not immune to the same kind of stressors that affect everyone else. Yet you also have the stress of being in pain and, perhaps, of wondering why you are in pain. If your pain is severe or has lasted a long time, you may have the stress of not being able to do the job you once did or of enjoying some sports or activities that once gave you pleasure. Sometimes, when you're aching, just the thought of having to get up from your bed or comfortable chair can be stressful!

Stress isn't always easy to deal with, but learning how to manage your stress can make it a little easier and help break the stress-pain-limited/lost abilities-depression cycle.

If stress is affecting your life and your health, learning to relax may be one of the most helpful things you can do for yourself, but you must understand that relaxing involves more than just kicking back and watching TV for an hour or two before bedtime. It requires that you become aware of what causes your stress and what you can do to eliminate the stressor or change your reaction to it.

For example, let's say that a major stressor in your life is dealing with the rush-hour commute to work and the toll the long car ride takes on your painful back. You could improve the situation by handling this stressor in one of two ways. First, you could try to eliminate the stressor. Some options:

- telecommuting (working from home and using computer and phone technology to do business or stay in touch with coworkers)
- changing your work hours to start and end during non-peak traffic times
- quitting your job and finding one closer to home or with different hours
  Second, you could change your responses to the stresses of rush-hour traffic. Some options for doing this:
- You could accept the fact that to keep your job you must drive in rush-hour traffic (no use getting upset about it).
- You could make the drive less stressful by leaving a little early to allow more time for delays, listening to upbeat music or audio books in the car, or practicing simple exercises to relieve stress and back pain when stopped at traffic lights.

As troublesome as stress is, something as simple as taking time to daydream or write in a journal can often help reduce your stress – and may even have beneficial effects on your pain and your disease.

Keeping a Stress Diary

An important first step to eliminating stress is to identify what causes it and how you respond both physically and emotionally. By keeping a simple stress diary daily, you should start to discover a pattern of stressors and symptoms. Then you can begin to address your stress using some of the techniques in this book. Here's an example you can follow:

Date	Time	Cause of Stress
11/10	5:00	Driving home in rush-hour traffic
11/19	6:35	Late picking up kids from day care, charged late fee, kids are upset
11/19	6:50-7:30	telemarketers call constantly while you try to prepare dinner
11/19	7:35	kids whine and act up at dinner table, spouse complains about meal
11/19	8:15-9:00	after-dinner clean-up and putting kids to bed as spouse lies on couch
11/19	11:00	trying to wind down, achy, unable to lie still enough to sleep while spouse snores loudly

Physical Symptoms	Emotional Symptoms
headache, heart beating faster, back aching	frustrated, anxious to get to kids' day care before closing
headache, heart racing, back aching more	guilt, frustration, anger
exhaustion, back aching	anger, irritation
growing fatigue	tension
growing tension in back	anger, feeling of hopelessness
achy, hot	frustration, irritation, anger

Relaxation Techniques

Relaxation techniques help you deal more calmly and effectively with life's stresses. Following are a few common techniques that might help:

Deep Breathing

To practice deep breathing, sit in a comfortable chair with your feet on the floor and your arms at your sides. Close your eyes and breathe in deeply, saying to yourself "I am…," then slowly out saying, "…relaxed."

Continue to breathe slowly, silently repeating something to yourself such as, "My hands …are warm; my feet …are warm; my breathing …is deep and smooth; my heartbeat …is calm and steady; I feel calm …and at peace."

Always coordinate the words with your breathing.

Distraction

Distraction involves training your mind to focus on something other than your stress or the sources of your stress. This does not mean that you will ignore your stress, only that you choose not to dwell on it.

When you anticipate a stressful situation, such as driving in heavy traffic or having to sit through a long office meeting, prepare yourself for the stress and how you will handle it. Make plans for what you will do once the stressful situation has passed, because even though it may seem at the time as if the problem will last forever, it will pass. By thinking of something else, you can take your mind off what is causing you stress.

Guided Imagery

Like distraction, guided imagery helps take your focus off your stress. To practice guided imagery, close your eyes, take a deep breath and hold in for several seconds. Breathe out slowly, feeling your body relax as you do.

Think about a place you have been where you felt safe and comfortable. Imagine it in as much detail as possible. Imagine the sounds you heard – of waves against the sand, seagulls calling overhead, children laughing on the beach. Imagine the way it felt, smelled and tasted – the saltwater on your lips, the soft sand beneath your feet, the ocean breeze blowing through your hair. Recapture the positive feelings you had when you were there and keep them in your mind. Take several deep breaths and enjoy feeling calm and peaceful before you open your eyes.

Progressive Relaxation

Progressive relaxation is a therapy in which the body's muscles, from head to toe, are progressively tensed and then relaxed. Progressive relaxation is a popular form of stress management.

To practice progressive relaxation, first close your eyes and take a deep breath, filling your chest, and breathe in all the way down to your abdomen. Breathe out, letting your stress flow out with the air. Beginning with your feet and calves, slowly tense your muscles. Hold for several seconds, then release and relax the muscles. Slowly work your way through your major muscle groups using the same technique, until you have tensed and relaxed the muscles of your neck and face. Continue breathing deeply and enjoy the feeling of relaxation before opening your eyes.

Visualization

One of the most stressful aspects of unrelenting back pain, or pain that comes and goes with no predictable pattern, is that it can make you feel as if your life is out of your control. **Visualization** helps reduce that stress by allowing you to imagine yourself anyway you like, doing anything you want to do. In other words, you are in control of the scenario. Also, by focusing on doing the things you like, you are not focusing on the things that cause you stress.

One form of visualization involves concentrating on pleasant scenes from your past or creating new situations in your mind. For example, you might try to remember every detail of a special vacation or your first date with your husband or wife. Alternatively, you could imagine yourself taking your dream vacation or having a date with an attractive movie star.

Another form of visualization involves thinking of symbols that represent the pain or stress in different parts of your body. For example, you might imagine that your painful lower back is bright red, then imagine yourself making the red fade or change to cool, soothing blue. You might imagine your pain as a little monster that you could put in a trash can and shut the lid. For some specific mental exercises to help you relax, try the following relaxation exercises.

Sample Relaxation Exercises

For the following exercises, you'll never have to break a sweat or even leave your easy chair, because your mind is doing the work. Pick a place where you won't be interrupted, get quiet and comfortable, and start to focus on your breathing. Imagine that fresh air is coming in and tension is being released with every breath. Then try one or more of the exercises described below. Pick a favorite exercise to save for times when you're feeling stressed.

Pain Drain

Feel within your body and note where you experience pain or tension. Imagine that the pain or tension is turning into a liquid substance. This heavy liquid flows down through your body and through your fingers and toes. Allow the pain to drain from your body in a steady flow. Now imagine that a gentle stream flows down over your head . . . and further dissolves the pain . . . into a liquid that continues to drain away. Enjoy the sense of comfort and well-being that follows.

Disappearing Pain

Notice any tension or pain that you are experiencing. Imagine that the pain takes the form of an object... or several objects. It can be fruit, pebbles, crystals or anything else that comes to mind. Pick up each piece of pain, one at a time, and place it in a magic box.

As you drop each piece into the box, it dissolves into nothingness. Now, again survey within your body to see if any pieces remain, and you may remove them if you wish. Imagine that your body is lighter now, and allow yourself to experience a feeling of comfort and well-being. Enjoy this feeling of tranquility and repose.

Healing Potion

Imagine you are in a drugstore that is stocked with bottles and jars of exotic potions. Each potion has a special magical quality. Some are pure white light, others are lotions, balms and creams, and yet others contain healing vibrations. As you survey the many potions, choose one that appeals to you. It may even have your name on the container. Open the container and cover your body with that magical potion. As you apply it, let any pain or tension slowly melt away, leaving you with a feeling of comfort and well-being. Imagine that you place the container in a special spot and that it continually renews its contents for future use.

BIOFEEDBACK

Imagine being able to lower your heart rate or blood pressure at will. Using a process called **biofeedback**, the idea is not as far-fetched as it sounds. In fact, biofeedback can help you control many body processes that previously were considered to be out of conscious control. Biofeedback also can help you control your body's response to stress.

What is biofeedback? In a nutshell, it's the use of electronic instruments to measure body functions and feed this information back to you so that you can learn to control them. With practice, you can learn to control almost any body process that can be measured.

In a biofeedback session, sensors are attached to the part of the body being monitored – such as your cold hands or a stiff muscle in your neck – and then connected to an electronic instrument, such as computer. The instruments might read your skin temperature, electrical signals produced by your muscles, your heart rate, or your brain waves. If the prospect of having sensors attached to you sounds frightening, it's not. Nor is it painful.

The practitioner conducting biofeedback will teach you some relaxation techniques, such as visualization (see page 155), to influence your subconscious body processes. As you practice these mental techniques, the instruments feed back the effects your thoughts are having on your body with sound, light or other signals. Eventually, you will learn what mental techniques to use to get the physical effect you want and you will be able to do them without the equipment.

KEEPING A JOURNAL

When you were an adolescent, you may have found that confiding in a diary or journal – about a fight with your best friend, exam-time anxiety or a breakup with your latest heartthrob, for example – helped defuse some of the emotions that came with a stressful or hurtful experience. Research shows that a variation on the writing you may have done then can help you cope with the stress that accompanies or contributes to pain now. For some people, keeping a journal may even help the problems underlying their back pain.

A recent study of people with rheumatoid arthritis showed that those who regularly wrote about their most stressful life events experienced a 28 percent reduction in overall disease activity. Although it was just a single study, it substantiates long-held speculation that stress can contribute to pain and disease activity. It also shows that reducing stress – specifically by writing about emotionally painful events – may actually decrease the severity of your pain.

At the very least, keeping a journal can help you identify situations that cause you stress, and identifying stressors is the first step to finding ways to cope with or eliminate them. On page 152, you'll find a sample stress diary that you can use as a model to get you started. If you prefer a more free-form approach, try some of the following suggestions to begin your journaling:

Choose your paper. Find a spiral notebook or blank book with lots of open space to begin writing.

Don't worry about penmanship or spelling. A journal should be for your eyes only, so you won't need to impress anyone with neat writing, proper grammar and expert spelling. Stopping to look up a word in the dictionary or contemplate grammatical issues can interfere with self-expression.

Choose the time and place. Don't try to write in your journal while you watch TV or stir a pot of soup on the stove. Pick a place without distractions and a time when you won't be interrupted. Focus entirely on your writing.

Don't hold back. Don't be afraid to express your emotions – all of them. Your journal won't judge you and no one else will have to see it.

Pick your style. You may wish to write about events as if you were a newspaper reporter covering your life, or you may wish to write your feelings in a letter – aren't there a few things you would like to tell your back pain? You may find one style that you'll want to stick with or you may vary your style from day to day. It's your book – do what works for you.

Get help if you need it. Writing can stir painful feelings, which may be difficult to deal with – that's part of the process of letting go of pain and stress. If you feel you need help coping with the feelings that writing arouses, consult a counselor or clergy member. Sometimes taking your journal along with you to counseling – and reading selected passages aloud – can help your counselor help you.

chapter 10

Back to You

By now you are aware that there are many, many things that can be done for back pain. Some of these, including surgery or prescription medication, require that you see a doctor. In fact, it's important that you consult a doctor or other health professional about any treatment you are considering – even therapies that don't require a prescription.

Beyond these therapies, the strategies you use to ease your back pain – and, therefore, the results you ultimately achieve – are largely up to you. As we learned in this book, it is vital that you become a good self-manager of your back pain. It's important that you take control of your pain by being an active participant in your ongoing care.

Ask yourself the following questions: Will you take the medication your doctor prescribes exactly as it is prescribed? Will you be faithful in doing the exercises to strengthen weak abdominal muscles? Will you write in a stress diary, practice relaxation techniques, prepare an ice pack or soak in a hot tub when you're in pain? Will you try a firmer mattress or more practical shoes? Will you stop smoking, cut down on fatty foods, remember your daily calcium tablet and be mindful of proper posture? When nothing else seems to help, will you try something new, perhaps a yoga class, self-massage or reflexology?

Only you can answer these questions. Only you can take the initiative to do what it takes to reduce your back pain. Your doctor can prescribe medication, but he or she can't watch you every day to be sure you remember to take it – and take the right amount. Your physical therapist can teach you exercises, but he or she can't force you to do them regularly once you leave the office. Your dietitian may recommend changes in eating habits that will help you lose weight to take stress off your back, but he or she can't buy your groceries or keep watch over your pantry. You can learn a hundred ways to ease your pain, but none of them can work without earnest effort from the most important person in your health-care team: you.

In this book, you have learned a lot of therapies and back-healthy habits that can help you. If your back pain is severe, long-lasting or accompanied by other symptoms, such as numbness or tingling in a leg, by all means see a doctor – soon. (To find out what type of doctor you might want or need to see, refer to page 20.)

On the other hand, if your back symptoms are those of simple sprain or muscle strain (the majority of them are), or if you have pain that hasn't been resolved through surgery or medication alone, now is the time to try a few approaches of your own. By self-managing your back pain, with the guidance and support of health-care professionals, you can make great strides toward a more active, healthy lifestyle.

In this final chapter, we will recap, in a series of brief checklists, many of the therapies featured in this book. Look over the lists to find the objectives you would like to achieve, then read on for tips and techniques for achieving them.

Use these lists to devise your own pain treatment plan (note that items often appear on more than one list), develop a repertoire of techniques to use when pain is at it worst and make healthy, conscious choices that add up to long-term pain relief and prevention.

To Make the Most of Your Medical Treatment

❏ Find a doctor you trust. For tips on selecting a doctor, see page 37.

❏ Don't insist on a diagnosis right away. Many times, the exact cause of back pain is not known, but your pain still can be treated successfully.

❏ Make sure you understand any medication you are taking – ask questions and check out "Understanding Medications: Where To Learn More" on page 56.

❏ Take your medications exactly as prescribed – no doubling doses when pain is severe.

❏ Question any doctor who insists on performing surgery; get a second opinion if you have doubts.

❏ Prepare well for surgery, if you choose to have it. For tips on preparing for surgery, see page 90.

❏ Always incorporate exercise and other healthy lifestyle habits into any prescribed treatment plan.

❏ Let your doctor know of any medication (including over-the-counter ones and nutritional supplements) you are taking. They may interact with the medicines he or she prescribes.

To Get Through a Painful Time

❏ Ask your physician about medication. You may need something stronger for unusual pain or medication to help you sleep.

- ❏ Soothe with heat – a hot water bottle, heating pad or warm bath.
- ❏ Cool the pain with commercial ice packs or with a plastic bag of ice cubes or frozen vegetables. (For tips on using heat and cold, see page 103.)
- ❏ Get enough rest, but not too much. More than a few days of bed rest can create more problems than it solves.
- ❏ Stay active if possible. For gentle exercises, see page 112.
- ❏ Try relaxation techniques. For specifics on how to use various techniques, see page 141.

To Make Exercise Less Painful

- ❏ Start slowly with exercise and build up gradually.
- ❏ Don't try to do specific back exercises during the first two weeks of an acute back pain episode.
- ❏ Try exercising in water. Most exercises that you can do on land, you can do in water – and with less pain.
- ❏ Check out new forms of exercise and movement therapies: yoga, tai chi, Alexander technique, Feldenkrais and Pilates.

To Build a Stronger Spine

- ❏ Have bone density tests if recommended by your doctor.
- ❏ Consume a diet rich in calcium.
- ❏ Take any bone-building medications exactly as prescribed.
- ❏ Take a daily calcium supplement and other supplements as recommended by your doctor or dietitian.
- ❏ Up your activity level. Any exercise helps; weight-bearing exercise is best.
- ❏ Avoid excessive alcohol and avoid smoking – period.

To Improve Lifestyle Choices
That Affect Your Back

❏ Pick more practical shoes. For shoe-buying tips, see page 124.

❏ Lose weight if necessary.

❏ Avoid high-fat foods that can affect the blood vessels in your back – and elsewhere.

❏ Stop smoking.

❏ Be mindful of your posture. (For specifics on how to sit and stand, see page 116.)

To Relieve Stress-Related
Pain Through Relaxation

❏ Get a massage – or give yourself one. (For how-to tips, see page 101).

❏ Listen to relaxing music.

❏ Take a warm bath.

❏ Use guided imagery, visualization, deep breathing or distraction. (See instructions for specific exercises and techniques, page 141.)

To Get a Good Night's Sleep

❏ Try taking an NSAID before bedtime.

❏ Try a firmer mattress or putting a piece of plywood under the one you have.

❏ Try to sleep on your side or back.

❏ Take a warm bath before bedtime.

❏ Get plenty of exercise – preferably early in the day.

❏ Follow these and other "Tips for Getting a Good Night Sleep" on page 12.

To Make the Most of Complementary Therapies

❏ Consult your doctor or other health-care professional about any therapy you are considering.

❏ Learn as much as you can about the therapy – read product labels and check out "Evaluating Alternative and Complementary Therapies" on page 148.

❏ Don't abandon a treatment that works. If your back pain results from an underlying disease, such as ankylosing spondylitis or rheumatoid arthritis, going off your prescribed treatment can be dangerous.

❏ Focus on pain relief. Pain is one of the symptoms most likely to respond to alternative and complementary therapies. Treatments you might want to try for pain relief include:

  – herbs and nutritional supplements

  – acupuncture

  – acupressure

To Prevent or Lessen Future Episodes of Pain

❏ Adopt back-healthy habits.

❏ Choose proper footwear.

❏ Strive for good posture.

❏ Avoid tobacco and excessive alcohol.

❏ Consume a healthy diet and maintain a proper weight.

❏ Get plenty of exercise. For specific exercises that can help your back, see page 112.

❏ Get plenty of sleep.

❑ Practice proper lifting techniques.

❑ Use a good, firm mattress (or reinforce your soft one, if it helps).

Although back pain is never pleasant, it doesn't have to be incapacitating or permanent. There is plenty that can be done to ease back pain and minimize its effects on your life, but the work begins and ends with you. The power to improve your back pain largely is in your hands.

We hope that this book has been an informative resource for you as you learn more about back pain, its causes, its treatments and its ongoing management and prevention. Refer to it often and always work closely with your health-care team as you find the treatments, techniques and solutions that work best for you.

With the information you have learned in this book, and the guidance that you can get from your doctor and other health-care professionals, you are now on the road to a healthier, less painful back. By taking an active role to control your back pain, you increase your chances of having a more active life as well. Don't let back pain control you – take control of your back pain.

GLOSSARY

A

Acupuncture – Eastern medicine technique in which thin needles are used to puncture the body at specific sites along energy pathways call meridians. Although still widely considered an alternative therapy, acupuncture is gaining acceptance in Western medicine, primarily for use in pain relief. *Acupressure* is another form of this treatment, but one involving hand pressure rather than needle punctures.

Acute pain – pain that comes on rapidly and lasts about one to seven days

Alexander technique – a therapy that teaches proper posture through mind-body awareness and helps you replace postural habits that contribute to pain with healthier habits

American Academy of Orthopaedic Surgeons (AAOS) – organization that provides educa-tion and practice management services for orthopaedic surgeons and allied health professionals. The Academy also serves as an advocate for improved patient care and informs the public about the science of orthopaedics. See *orthopaedist*.

American College of Rheum-atology – the professional organi-zation of rheumatologists, doctors who specialize in diagnosing and treating rheumatic diseases. See *rheumatologist*.

Analgesic – a medication used to relieve pain

Ankylosing spondylitis (AS) – a form of arthritis that mainly affects the spine and sacroiliac joints (where the spine attaches to the pelvis). In severe cases, AS may cause the spine to become fused and rigid.

Arachnoiditis – scarring of tissue surrounding the spinal nerve roots (where the nerves exit the spine between the vertebrae) that can cause pain, numbness and tingling in the legs. The most common cause is scarring from prior back surgery.

B

Back – the part of the body spanning from the back of the neck to the buttocks that consists of the spine and its supporting tissues, including muscles, tendons and ligaments

Biofeedback – the use of electronic instruments to measure body functions and feed that information back to you, allowing you to learn how to control body processes, such as heart rate or blood pressure, that are generally thought to be out of conscious control

Bisphosphonates – a class of medications that inhibit bone resorption and are used to treat bone diseases such as osteoporosis

C

Capsaicin – a pain-relieving substance derived from cayenne pepper that is the active ingredient in some analgesic rubs

Cauda equina syndrome – a condition in which the nerve roots that supply the bladder and bowel, along with the groin and anal areas, are compressed. This compression leads to loss of sensation and sexual function and an inability to urinate. Without surgery to relieve compression on these nerve roots, the condition could become permanent.

Cervical spine – the neck and upper back, composed of the seven vertebrae closest to the skull

GLOSSARY

Charley horse – a painful cramp in the leg muscles, particularly the calf muscle

Chiropractic – practice of healing based on spinal manipulation and the belief that illness stems from malalignment of the spinal cord. See *chiropractor*.

Chiropractor – a health practitioner who is trained and licensed to practice *chiropractic*, a widely used therapy that focuses on the manual adjustment of the spine to relieve pain and disease

Chronic pain – long-term pain that lasts more than three months

Coccyx – the lower-most segment of the spine, composed of four fused vertebrae; also referred to as the tailbone

Coccydynia – literally translated "pain in the coccyx (tailbone)." Coccydynia is usually the result of trauma, such as falling directly onto your buttocks.

COX-2 specific inhibitor – a type of nonsteroidal anti-inflammatory drug (NSAID) that is designed to be safer for the stomach than other NSAIDs. COX-2 inhibitors work by inhibiting hormone-like substances in the body that cause pain and inflammation without interfering with similar substances that protect the stomach lining.

CT Scan – short for computerized tomography, a diagnostic test that involves using a computer to record two-dimensional "slice" images of your body and then turning those slices into a three-dimensional view of the back. Also known as *CAT Scan*.

D

DEXA – short for dual-energy X-ray absorptiometry, a scan that measures bone density at the hip and spine to diagnose osteoporosis and evaluate bone density

Disc – small, circular cushions positioned between the vertebrae in the spine. Each disc consists of two parts: a strong outer cover called the annulus fibrosis, and a "jelly filling" called the nucleus pulposis.

Discectomy – the surgical removal of part of a disc that is herniated and causing pain. The majority of discectomies performed in this country are referred to as either percutaneous (through the skin) or microsurgical.

Discitis – inflammation of the discs, which is rare and typically caused by infection

Discogram – a test used to view and assess the internal structure of a disc (the crescent-shaped pieces of connective tissue located between the vertebrae) and to determine if the disc is a source of pain

DISH – short for diffuse idiopathic skeletal hypertosis, a disorder that causes excess bone to grow between the vertebrae, most commonly of the neck and lower back, which results in stiffness

DMARDs – short for disease-modifying antirheumatic drugs, a class of medications that work to modify the course of rheumatoid arthritis and other forms of inflammatory arthritis, slowing or even stopping its progression

E

Elective surgery – surgery performed for any reason other than imminent

GLOSSARY

risk to health or life. Most back surgeries are considered elective.

Epidural anesthesia – anesthetic injected directly into the spinal canal, between the spinal column and the outermost cover of the spinal cord. Epidural anesthesia is used to numb the lower half of the body during surgery.

Epidural steroid injection – a treatment for back pain that involves injecting a glucocorticoid compound directly into the epidural space (the area between the spinal column and outermost cover of the spinal cord) to relieve localized inflammation.

Erythrocyte sedimentation rate (ESR) – Also referred to as *sed rate*, a test measuring how fast red blood cells (erythrocytes) clump together and fall to the bottom of a test tube like sediment. A high (fast) sedimentation rate signals the presence of inflammation, possibly indicating an inflammatory disease such as rheumatoid arthritis.

Facet joints – the connection points between the vertebrae. These joints keep the spine aligned as it moves.

Facet joint block – a procedure in which a steroid and/or anesthetic medication is injected directly into the facet joint capsule. The procedure is used both in diagnosis, to determine the source of back pain, and in treatment of pain resulting from injuries to the facet joints.

Facet neurotomy – a treatment for back pain that involves using a probe heated with radio waves to disable a nerve that is supplying an injured facet joint.

Facet syndrome – an inflammation of one or more of the facet joints where the vertebrae connect to one another

Fatigue – a generalized, long-lasting feeling of tiredness or sleepiness that isn't relieved by sleep or rest

Feldenkrais method – a program of more than a thousand different movements designed to increase body awareness, flexibility and range of motion. Feldenkrais practitioners use a combination of these movements, along with hands-on manipulations, to gradually teach the body to work more efficiently.

Fibromyalgia – an arthritis-related syndrome characterized by widespread muscle pain, the presence of tender points (or points on the body that feel painful on pressure) and often debilitating fatigue and other symptoms.

G

Glucocorticoids – a group of hormones, including cortisol, produced by the adrenal glands. They can be synthetically produced (that is, made in a laboratory) and have powerful anti-inflammatory effects. These drugs include prednisone and are sometimes called *corticosteroids* or *steroids*.

H

Herniated discs – also referred to as *ruptured discs*, a painful condition that occurs when discs are injured and their jelly-like center leaks out through the tough outer coating, causing irritation to nearby nerves

I

Inflammation – an immune-system response to injury or infection that causes heat, redness and swelling

GLOSSARY

in the affected area. Inflammation is a common cause of pain, such as in injury or arthritis. In some forms of arthritis, joint and organ inflammation occurs as a result of a faulty immune response to the body's own tissues.

Internist – a doctor who specializes in the diagnosis, prevention and treatment of all forms of adult disease. Training for an internist requires four years of medical school, followed by a three-year in-hospital residency. Internists may choose to take additional subspecialty training in particular fields, such as rheumatology, endocrinology, cardiology or gastroenterology.

K

Kyphosis – an abnormal forward curvature of the upper spine. Sometimes referred to as *hunchback* or a *dowager's hump*.

L

Lamina – the lining of the hole (spinal canal) in the vertebrae through which the spinal cord runs. See *spinal cord*.

Laminectomy – the surgical removal of the back of the spinal canal that forms a roof over the spinal cord. The purpose of the procedure is to relieve pain by enlarging the spinal column to make more room for nerves that have become compressed within the column.

Ligaments – tough bands of connective tissue that attach bones to bones and help keep them together at a joint

Lumbar spine – the lower back, composed of five vertebrae

M

MRI – short for magnetic resonance imaging, MRI is a procedure in which a very strong magnet is used to pass a force through the body to create a clear, detailed image of a cross-section of the body.

Muscle – fibrous tissue in the body that holds us upright and gives the body movement, including movement that we consciously initiate (such as waving a hand) and movement of which we are scarcely aware (such as movement of the blood through the vessels or food through the digestive system).

N

Narcotic – a type of analgesic medication used to relieve severe pain by depressing brain function. The name is used particularly for morphine and other derivatives of opium. See *analgesic*.

Neurologist – a doctor who has advanced training in diagnosing and treating problems related to the nervous system

Neurosurgeon – a doctor who has specialty training in the surgical treatment of problems related to the nervous system

Nonsteroidal anti-inflammatory drugs (NSAIDs) – a class of medications commonly used to ease the pain and inflammation of many forms of arthritis, including aspirin, ibuprofen and naproxen

Nurse or nurse practitioner – a person who has received education and training in health care, particularly patient care. Many nurses have earned a registered nurse degree, noted by an RN in

GLOSSARY

their title. *Nurse practitioners* are registered nurses with advanced training and emphasis in primary care, who can diagnose illness and, in many states, prescribe medication.

O

Orthopaedic surgeon – a doctor who specializes in surgery involving the musculoskeletal system, including the bones and joints

Orthopaedist – a medical doctor who specializes in treatment (largely through surgery) of problems involving the musculoskeletal system, including the bones and joints. This term often is used interchangeably with orthopaedic surgeon.

Ossify – to develop into bone

Osteoarthritis (OA) – the most common form of arthritis. OA causes cartilage breakdown at certain joints (including the spine, hands, hips and knees), resulting in pain and deformity.

Osteopathy – a system of medicine emphasizing body mechanics along with more traditional treatment and diagnostic methods

Osteoporosis – a condition in which the body loses so much bone mass that bones are susceptible to disabling fractures under the slightest trauma

P

Paget's disease – a disease in which bone breaks down excessively and then is reformed abnormally. As a result, bones may be large but weak.

Physical therapist (PT) – a licensed health-care professional who specializes in using exercise to treat medical conditions. A PT also may prescribe canes, braces and splints, and some are trained in massage.

Physiatrist – a medical doctor who specializes in problems of the muscles and bones. Physiatrists typically focus on a non-medication rehabilitation approach to back pain.

Placebo effect – the phenomenon in which a person receiving an inactive drug or therapy experiences a reduction in symptoms

Prolotherapy – also called *sclerotherapy*, *regenerative injection therapy* or *nonsurgical ligament reconstruction*, a therapy in which a dextrose, or sugar, solution is injected directly into damaged back tissues. The theory is that the solution acts as an irritant to cause an inflammatory process that will increase blood flow to and, thus, healing of the injured tissue.

Q

Qi – an essential life energy that flows through the body along invisible channels called meridians, according to ancient Chinese beliefs. An imbalance of qi supposedly is the source of health problems and the balance can be restored through acupuncture. See *acupuncture*.

R

Rheumatoid arthritis – a chronic inflammatory form of arthritis in which the body's otherwise protective immune system turns against the body and attacks tissues of the joints, causing pain, inflammation and deformity

GLOSSARY

S

Sacroiliac – the joints where the spine attaches to the pelvis

Sacrum – the base of the spine, composed of five fused vertebrae, that attaches to the pelvis

Salicylates – a subcategory of nonsteroidal anti-inflammatory drugs (NSAIDs) that contain salicylates, which includes aspirin; also describes topical creams that relieve pain and inflammation. See *NSAIDs*.

Scoliosis – a condition in which the spine twists to one side. Scoliosis can be classified as true (meaning it has to do with abnormal development of the spine) or functional (meaning its cause is not directly related to the spine).

Selective nerve-root block – an injection of a steroid and/or numbing agent into the area of the nerve where it exits the spinal column between the vertebrae. The procedure is used in diagnosis, to determine the source of pain, and in treatment of back and leg pain, particularly that which results from a herniated disc.

SERMs (selective estrogen receptor molecules) – a class of osteoporosis medications that work much like estrogen to slow bone loss, but lack estrogen's side effects on uterine and breast tissues

Spasm – painful, involuntary contractions of the muscles

Spinal stenosis – "spinal narrowing." Spinal stenosis can occur when bone overgrowth of the spine causes the spinal column to narrow and press on the nerves housed within.

Spinal cord – the bundle of nerves that runs through the spinal column from the base of the spine to the brain. The spinal cord relays signals between the brain and all parts of the body via 31 pairs of smaller nerve bundles that branch off the spinal cord and exit the column between the vertebrae.

Spinal fusion – a surgical welding process by which two or more vertebrae are fused together to form a single immobile unit

Spinous process – the bony protrusions (bumps) in the spine you feel when you run your hand down your back

Spondyloarthropathies – a group of arthritis-related diseases that primarily affect the spine, including ankylosing spondylitis

Spondylolisthesis – a painful condition of the spine that results when a vertebra moves out of place and pinches a nerve

Spondylolysis – a painful condition in which the vertebrae of the spine detach from one another because of weak or damaged facet joints

Sprain – damage to ligaments, which in severe cases, can result in a complete tear of the structure

Spurs – sharp bony projections, such as those that may result from osteoarthritic changes in the spine

Strain – painful damage to the muscles that can occur with excessive use or stretching of poorly conditioned muscles. Muscle strain is the most common mechanical cause of back pain.

GLOSSARY

Subacute pain – pain that lasts between seven days and seven weeks and is typically mild. See *acute pain*.

T

Tai chi – an ancient Chinese practice that involves gentle, fluid movements and meditation to help strengthen muscles, improve balance and relieve stress

Tender points – specific, precise areas on the body that are particularly painful upon the application of slight pressure. The finding of tender points is useful in the diagnosis of fibromyalgia.

TENS – a treatment for pain that uses a small device to direct mild electric pulses to nerves in the painful area

Thoracic spine – the middle back, made up of the 12 vertebrae between the cervical and lumbar spine

Traction – the use of pulleys, weights and other devices to pull the upper and lower parts of the body in opposite directions to open space between the vertebrae. In back pain, traction is used to relieve pressure on discs.

Transverse processes – a pair of protrusions on either side of the vertebrae to which the back muscles attach. See *spinous process*.

Trigger points – points on the body that trigger pain elsewhere in the body when pressure is applied to them

V

Vertebrae – the individual bones that are stacked one on top of another to form the spinal column

Whiplash – damage to the ligaments, vertebrae, spinal cord or nerve roots in the upper (cervical) spine, caused by a sudden jerking back of the head and neck

Yoga – an ancient Indian practice that involves a series of body postures and includes exercise, meditation and breathing components to improve posture and balance and help relieve stress on the joints, as well as emotional stress

About the Arthritis Foundation

PROGRAMS, SERVICES AND INFORMATIONAL RESOURCES TO HELP YOU TAKE CONTROL

This book is published by the Arthritis Foundation, the only national, voluntary health organization working for the more than 43 million Americans with arthritis or related diseases. The Arthritis Foundation offers many valuable resources through more than 150 offices nationwide. The chapter that serves your area has information, products, classes and other services to put you in charge of your arthritis. To find the office near you, call 800/283-7800 or search the Arthritis Foundation Web site at www.arthritis.org.

Programs and Services

Physician referral – Most Arthritis Foundation chapters can provide a list of doctors in your area who specialize in the evaluation and treatment of arthritis and arthritis-related diseases.

Exercise programs – The Arthritis Foundation sponsors, develops and coordinates exercise programs for people with arthritis, featuring specially-trained instructors. They include:

PACE (People with Arthritis Can Exercise) – These courses feature gentle movements to increase joint flexibility, range of motion, stamina and muscle strength. An accompanying video is available for home use.

Arthritis Foundation Aquatic Program – These water exercise programs help relieve strain on muscles and joints. An accompanying PEP (Pool Exercise Program) video is available for home use. This program is taught at many YMCAs around the country, where it is called AFYAP (Arthritis Foundation YMCA Aquatic Program).

Educational and Self-Help Groups – The Arthritis Foundation sponsors mutual-support groups that provide opportunities for discussion and problem-solving among people with arthritis. In addition, the Arthritis Foundation offers courses designed to help people actively manage their particular disease through exercise, medications, relaxation techniques, pain management, nutrition and more. These include the Arthritis Self-Help Course and the Fibromyalgia Self-Help Course.

Information and Products

Find the latest information about arthritis, including research, medications, government advocacy, programs and services through one of the many information resources offered by the Arthritis Foundation:

www.arthritis.org – Information about arthritis is available 24 hours a day on the Internet at the Arthritis Foundation's interactive, comprehensive Web site. Find news about arthritis, ways to get involved, and a variety of useful arthritis products, including books, brochures, videos and more. In addition, the Arthritis Foundation has a new interactive self-management guide for people with arthritis, *Connect and Control: Your Online Arthritis Action Guide*. Via questionnaire responses, *Connect and Control* helps participants create a customized self-management program for their unique challenges, including tailored information on pain management, joint protection, fitness, diet and more.

Arthritis Answers – Call toll-free at 800/283-7800 for 24-hour, automated information about arthritis and Arthritis Foundation resources. Trained volunteers and staff are also available at your local Arthritis Foundation chapter to answer questions or refer you to physicians and other resources. For general questions about arthritis, you can also call 404-872-7100 ext. 1, or email questions to help@arthritis.org.

Publications

The Arthritis Foundation offers many publications to educate people with arthritis, as well as their families and friends, about diagnosis, medications, exercise, diet, pain management and more.

Books – The Arthritis Foundation publishes a variety of books on arthritis to help you learn to understand and manage your condition, live a healthier life, and cope with the emotional challenges that come with a chronic illness. Order books directly at www.arthritis.org or by calling 800/207-8633. All Arthritis Foundation books are available at your local bookstore.

Brochures – The Arthritis Foundation offers brochures containing concise, understandable information on the many arthritis-related diseases and conditions, including back pain. Topics include surgery, the latest medications, guidance for working with your doctors, ways to improve your fitness and flexibility, and self-managing your illness. Several brochures are also available in Spanish. Single copies are available free of charge at www.arthritis.org or by calling 800/283-7800.

Arthritis Today – This award-winning bimonthly magazine provides the latest information on research, new treatments, trends and tips from experts and readers to help you manage arthritis. A one-year subscription to *Arthritis Today* is included when you become a member of the Arthritis Foundation. Annual membership is $20 and helps fund research to find cures for arthritis. Call 800/933-0032 for information.

Kids Get Arthritis Too – This newsletter focusing on juvenile rheumatic diseases, is published six times a year. Features speak to children and teens with the illness as well as to their parents. Stories examine the latest news in diagnosis, treatment and research of children's rheumatic diseases, as well as helpful ways kids can cope with their illnesses and the challenges they bring. This newsletter is now a free benefit of membership in the Arthritis Foundation and can be ordered when you join. Call 800/933-0032 for information.

Videos – The Arthritis Foundation produces several videos designed to increase your fitness without putting undue strain on your muscles, back and joints from injury. The PACE (People with Arthritis Can Exercise) video series instructs the viewer in exercises people of any ability level can perform. Also available are the Fibromyalgia Interval Training (FIT) and Pool Exercise Program (PEP) exercise videos, and a Spanish-language video, Senderos Para Vivir Mejor con la Artritis (Pathways to Better Living With Arthritis). Visit www.arthritis.org or call 800/207-8633 to order.

Research and Advocacy

The Arthritis Foundation is the second largest funding source for arthritis research, behind the National Institutes of Health (NIH). Since its inception in 1948, the Arthritis Foundation has invested more than $244 million on research, including both basic and clinical research targeted at better understanding various forms of arthritis and related conditions and improving treatment for people with them.

The Foundation is also involved in numerous advocacy issues, from working to increase funding for arthritis research by the federal government to ensuring access to care. To learn how you can be advocate for people with arthritis and play a role in forming public policy, call your local Arthritis Foundation office.

To find out more about the Arthritis Foundation's many efforts on behalf of people with arthritis and related diseases, or to donate to the Foundation's many causes, call your local chapter. Or, you may call 800/283-7800 or log on to www.arthritis.org.

Index

A

Acetaminophen (*Tylenol*), 41, 44–45

Acetaminophen with codeine (*Fioricet, Phenaphen* with *Codeine, Tylenol* with *Codeine*), 45

Acupoints, 142

Acupressure, 141, 143

Acupuncture, 141, 142–143, 170

Acute pain, 14, 170

Advil, 47

Aerobic exercises, 110

Alendronate (*Fosamax*), 55

Alexander technique, 139, 170

Alternative therapies. *See* Complementary and alternative therapies

American Academy of Family Physicians, 21

American Academy of Musculo-Skeletal Medicine, 68

American Academy of Neurology, 22

American Academy of Orthopaedic Surgeons (AAOS), 23, 170

American Academy of Physical Medicine and Rehabilitation, 21

American Association of Orthopaedic Medicine, 68

American College of Rheumatology, 21, 170

American Osteopathic Association, 22

Amitriptyline (*Elavil*), 51

Analgesics, 44–47, 170
  narcotic, 45
  topical, 45–47

Anesthesia for back surgery, 92–94
  epidural, 93
  general, 93
  local, 93
  regional, 93

Angry cat stretch, 115

Ankylosing spondylitis (AS), 170
  complete blood count in diagnosing, 35
  diet and, 122
  as form of arthritis, 8
  massage therapy for, 101
  medications for, 52
  symptoms of, 33
  tumor necrosis factor in, 53–54

Annulus fibrosis, 3

Anterior longitudinal ligament, 5

Antidepressants, 51

Aortic aneurysms as cause of back pain, 13

Arachnoiditis, 12, 171

ArthriCare, 46

Arthritis, 7, 8–9
  with inflammatory bowel disease, 9
  medications for, 52–54
  psoriatic, 9
  reactive, 9, 52
  rheumatoid, 9

Arthritis Foundation, 58
  aquatics program, 111, 185
  educational and support groups, 185
  information and products, 185–186
  PACE, 184
  programs and services, 184–185
  publications, 186–188
  research and advocacy, 188–189

Arthritis Foundation's Guide to Alternative Therapies, 148

Arthritis Today's Drug Guide, 58

Arthrotec, 50

Asanas, 137

Aspercreme, 46

Copper, 132
Corsets, 105
Counterirritants, 46
Crab shells, 131
Crunches, 114
Cyclobenzaprine (*Flexeril*), 51
Cyclooxygenase-2 (COX-2)
    inhibitors, 48, 49, 172
Cytokines, 53

D

Deep breathing, 154
Degenerative disc disease, 5–6, 6, 68
Depression as cause of back pain, 13
Devil's claw, 130
Diagnosis
    blood tests in, 34–35
    dual energy X-ray
        absorptiometry in, 31
    facet joint blocks in, 65
    imaging tests in, 27–31
    medical history in, 23–24
    medical tests in, 27–37
    nerve tests in, 31–32, 34–35
    physical exam in, 24–26
    psychological tests in, 35, 37
    sacroiliac joint blocks in, 67
    selective nerve root block in, 63
Diet and weight management, 121–123
Dietary supplements, 128
Diffuse idiopathic skeletal
    hyperostosis (DISH), 11, 173
Dihydrochloride, 46
Discectomy, 78–80, 173
    microsurgical, 79–80
    percutaneous, 78–80
Discitis, 12, 173
Discogram, 30–31, 173
Discs, 3, 173
    herniated, 6–7, 32, 175
    back surgery for, 77

ruptured, 6–7
Disease-modifying antirheumatic drugs
    (DMARDs), 52, 53, 173
Disease-related causes of
    back pain, 7–12
    arthritis, 8–9
    diffuse idiopathic skeletal hypertosis, 11
    fibromyalgia, 12
    infections, 12
    kyphosis, 11
    osteoporosis, 9–10
    Paget's disease, 11
    scoliosis, 11
    spinal stenosis, 10–11
    spondylolysis, 12
    tumors, 12
Distraction, 154
Docosahexaenoic acid (DHA), 133
Doctor
    identifying specialist, 20–23
    information for, 25
    working with, to find the
        right fit, 37–38
Double knee pull, 115
Dowager's hump, 11
Dual emission X-ray absorptiometry
    (DEXA), 31, 173

E

Effective self-manager, 96–97
Elective surgery, 173–174
Electroacupuncture, 142
Electrodiagnostic studies, 31
Electromyography (EMG), 34
Emotions, role of, in your pain, 75
Endometriosis as cause of back pain, 13
Endurance exercises, 110
Enzyme, 132
Epidural anesthesia, 93, 174
Epidural steroid injections, 62–63, 174
    risk of, 70

Erythrocyte sedimentation rate
  (ESR or "sed rate"), 35, 174
Esomeprazole magnesium (*Nexium*), 50
Estratab, 55
Estrogen, 55
Etanercept (*Enbrel*), 53
Eucalyptamint, 46
Eucalyptus oil, 46
Exercises, 108–115
  aerobic, 110
  endurance, 110
  isokinetic, 109–110
  isometric, 109
  isotonic, 109
  on land, 114–115
  making less painful, 165
  range-of-motion, 109
  relaxation, 156–157
  strengthening, 109
  in water, 110–113
  yoga, 137
Extensors, 5
Extracts, 129

F

Facet joint block, 174
Facet joints, 3, 64, 174
Facet neurotomy, 66, 174
Facets, 3
Facet syndrome, 7, 175
Failed back syndrome, 61
Famotidine (*Pepcid*), 50
Fatigue, 175
Feldenkrais method, 139–140, 175
Fibromyalgia, 12, 32, 175
  exam for, 36
Fish oil, 133
Flexall, 46
Flexors, 5

Fluoroscopy
  for epidural steroid injection, 63
  for facet joint blocks, 65
  for facet neurotomy, 66–67
  for percutaneous discectomy, 78
  for sacroiliac joint block, 67
Food Guide Pyramid, USDA, 121–122
Footwear, 124
Forward arm stretch, 113
Fracture, compression, 9–10, 83
Fractured vertebra, 33

G

Gabapentin (*Neurotonin*), 52
General anesthesia, 93
Ginger, 130
Glucocorticoid-induced osteoporosis, 56
Glucocorticoids, 86, 175
Glucosamine, 133
Guided imagery, 154–155

H

Hands-on therapies, 144–147
Herbal remedies, 128–130
Herb teas, 128
Herniated discs, 6–7, 32, 175
  back surgery for, 77
Histamine blockers (H2 blockers), 50
HLA-B27, 35
Hormones, 54–55
Hot and cold treatments, 102–103
Hot tubs
  exercises in, 113
  safety tips for, 99
Hunchback, 11
Hydrocodone with
  acetaminophen (*Ultracet*), 45
Hydroxychloroquine sulfate
  (*Plaquenil*), 53

Tender points, 26, 182
Therapeutic Mineral Ice, 46
Thoracic spine, 4, 182
Tinctures, 129
Tissue typing, 35
Tizanidine (*Zanaflex*), 52
Tobacco use, 124–125
Topical analgesics, 45–47
Traction, 182
Tramadol (*Ultram*), 45
Transcutaneous electrical
    nerve stimulation (TENS), 106, 182
Transverse processes, 3, 182
Trigger point injections, 69–70
Trigger points, 26, 69, 182
Tumor necrosis factor (TNF), 53–54
Tumors
    as cause of back pain, 12
    need for back surgery with, 88
Turpentine oil, 46

U

Ulcers, risk factors for, 48
Ultrasound, 104–105
United States Pharmacopoeia
    Dispensing Information (USPDI)
        Volume II Advice for the Patient,
        Drug Information in Lay
        Language, 57

V

Valdecoxib (*Bextra*), 48, 49
Vertebrae, 2, 15, 182
Vertebroplasty, 83–84
Visualization, 155–156, 158
Vitamins, 130–131
    B3, 131
    C, 131
    D, 131, 135
    E, 131

W

Walking, 117
Water, exercise in, 110–113
Water therapy, 98–99
Water walking, 112
Web sites, 57–58
Weight
    back surgery and, 86–87
    management of, 121–123
Wet tap, 61
Whiplash, 68, 183
Whole herbs, 128

X

X-rays in diagnosing, 27, 28

Y

Yoga, 137, 183

Z

Zanaflex, 52
Zantac, 50
Zostrix, 46

Get the Most Out of Life!

ONLY $24.95

TO ORDER, VISIT
www.arthritis.org

Please mention this code
when ordering: AFJF02A1
Item #835-245

CREATE A MORE HEALTHY, FULFILLING FUTURE.

The Arthritis Foundation's new **Guide to Managing Your Arthritis** gives you all the information you need to make the most of every day. This easy-to-understand book helps you manage pain, reduce stress, work with your health-care team and make sense of drugs, surgery and supplements. You'll learn simple exercises to help you ease stiffness and feel more mobile. Whether you are new to arthritis or have lived with it for years, this book has life-enhancing strategies for you.

Get the tools you need to create a more active, fulfilling life!

TO ORDER, CALL TOLL FREE
1-800-207-8633 (M-F 8:00 a.m. – 5:00 p.m. EST)

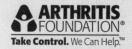

MYABKP2002